"I feel so much healthier and have more energy to play with my two lovely young grandchildren. After all those years, I no longer feel guilty about food: I'm in control."
Val Cornall, 50

"My GP told me I was one of those people who was destined to be fat. Then I tried the 8-Week Blood Sugar Diet. It's completely changed my life."
Sharon Pannett, 49

"I'd tried to lose weight over the years, but nothing seemed to work. Then I read about the 8-Week Blood Sugar Diet and threw myself into it. The effects were almost instant. I lost half a stone in the first week and my blood sugar readings dropped. At last, I felt like I could beat diabetes..."
Dawn Peace, 46

"It makes me sad to think I spent all those years being fat. And now, at last, I have the energy to live my life to the full." Jackie Lea-Bridges, 50

the
8-week
blood sugar
diet

the
8-week
blood sugar
diet

**Lose weight fast and
reprogramme your body**

DR MICHAEL MOSLEY

Published in the United Kingdom
in 2015 by Short Books,
Unit 316, ScreenWorks, 22 Highbury Grove,
London N5 2ER

36

A CIP catalogue record for this book
is available from the British Library.

ISBN: 978-1-78072-240-5

Recipes copyright © Dr Sarah Schenker
Photographs copyright © Romas Foord

Cover design by Andrew Smith
Printed at CPI Group (UK) Ltd, Croydon CR0 4YY

CONTENTS

THE SCIENCE

THE DIET

RECIPES AND MENU PLANS

FOREWORD

In 2006 I was turning the pages of a scientific journal when one particular page leapt out at me. It was reporting a study of weight loss (bariatric) surgery carried out on obese people with type 2 diabetes. The page showed a graph of the participants' blood sugar levels following the surgery. Within days of the operation, their blood sugar levels had returned to normal and many were able to come off their medication.

This was a striking finding because it was believed that type 2 diabetes was a lifelong, irreversible disease. People are usually advised that they have a condition which requires first tablets, then possibly insulin, and they must get used to living with diabetes.

But the reason this particular study grabbed my attention was that the return to normal blood sugar levels was so rapid. This fitted in with a theory I was developing at the time: that type 2 diabetes is simply the result of too much fat in the liver and pancreas interfering with insulin production. The sudden return to normal blood sugars had nothing to do with the surgery itself, but merely that eating had suddenly been cut down. If this theory was right, type 2 diabetes should be able to be completely reversed by food restriction alone.

Science moves slowly and carefully. Any hypothesis has to be tested rigorously. Over the last decade my research team and others working at Newcastle University have been investigating, in detail, the underlying mechanisms behind type 2 diabetes. We have developed new ways of measuring fat inside the liver and pancreas using powerful magnetic resonance scanners.

Now we have completed careful studies which have shown that people who really want to get rid of their type 2 diabetes can, in just 8 weeks, lose substantial amounts of weight and return blood sugar to normal or near normal. They remain free of diabetes provided they keep the weight off. We have shown that it is possible to reverse a disease that is still widely seen as irreversible.

So what is the long-term impact on overall health? Are there drawbacks for some people? To answer these and other important questions Diabetes UK has funded a large study in primary care which will run until 2018.

In the meantime I am delighted that Dr Michael Mosley is highlighting the importance of using weight loss to control blood sugar levels. His great skill is in communicating medical science and relating this to everyday life.

In this book about the biggest health problem of our time he pulls together hard scientific information from reliable sources, and weaves a tapestry which conveys great depth of understanding illustrated by many individual stories.

If you have type 2 diabetes and are interested in trying to regain full health, this is a book for you. If the condition runs in your family, then pass it round the family. In the 21st century we individually have to counteract a phenomenon new to our society: for the first time in 200,000 years of homo sapiens' evolution we need to learn how to avoid harm from the ever-present excess of food.

Prof Roy Taylor
November 2015

INTRODUCTION

Medicine and nutrition are areas where it often seems that the "truth" is constantly changing. New studies come along, sometimes reinforcing and sometimes undermining established wisdom. One moment fat is bad for you, the next it's good. The problem is that unless you keep up with the latest research, and are able to critically appraise it, you may end up feeling very confused. Hence this updated book, in which I have included some of the most recent studies and success stories.

It has been a year since I wrote the first edition of *The 8 week Blood Sugar Diet*, a book which, like my previous book *The Fast Diet*, has gone on to become an international bestseller.

I originally developed the book to help people, like me, who had been diagnosed with type 2 diabetes, or who were at risk of diabetes, and wanted to use diet rather than drugs to slow or even reverse the progression of their disease. I realised it had the added attraction of helping anyone who wanted to lose weight, fast, to do so, but I didn't realise how utterly life-changing it would be for so many.

Over the last year there have been even more studies

showing how adopting a low-carbohydrate Mediter-ranean-style way of eating is one of the best ways to combat a range of different conditions. More on that in Chapter six.

Results from a huge study, the largest of its kind ever undertaken, back up claims I make in this book that a rapid weight loss can be the best way to stem the apparently inexorable rise of type 2 diabetes. See Chapter five.

In early 2016 I also set up a website (thebloodsugardiet. com) where people share their experiences and offer helpful advice and tips. Heather, a mother of five, who had prediabetes, contacted me to say she had managed to lose an impressive 24lb in eight weeks and return her blood sugars to normal. "It's nothing short of a miracle."

Others, like Sharon, 49, who has been using steroid creams to treat severe eczema on her arms and trunk since she was a child, found that after a short while on The 8-Week Blood Sugar Diet she not only lost lots of weight but her eczema cleared. She also no longer needs the anti-inflammatory medicines she was taking for severe pain in her feet. "It's completely changed my life."

I've also been contacted by women who have found that doing this diet has helped them get rid of polycystic ovarian syndrome (PCOS) — a condition that affects one in five women and can make getting pregnant difficult.

Cassie, who you'll meet on page 75, not only managed to lose 44lb and reverse her PCOS, but got pregnant after years of trying. I am delighted to say she has recently given birth to a pair of lovely girls. "I'm 100 per cent certain I have these little girls only because of the diet."

I hope you enjoy this updated book and look forward to hearing more from you.

THE BLOOD SUGAR CRISIS

Millions of us have high blood sugar levels – and many of us don't know it.

Maybe you're often thirsty or need to urinate frequently. Perhaps you have cuts that are slow to heal or you are unusually tired. Or, far more likely, you have no symptoms at all.

Yet raised blood sugar is very bad news. It speeds up the ageing process, leads to type 2 diabetes and increases your risk of heart disease and stroke.

This is a book about blood sugar. It is about the epidemic of type 2 diabetes that has engulfed the world in recent years. It is also about the insidious build-up of blood sugar that precedes type 2 diabetes – a condition known as prediabetes. This is a wake-up call. A warning.

But there's no point in highlighting a problem unless you can do something about it. So if you have type 2 diabetes I am going to introduce you to a diet that in just eight weeks can reverse it. If you have prediabetes, I will show you how to stop it progressing.

Why do I care? Because a few years ago I was diagnosed as a type 2 diabetic; my blood sugar was out of control.

First, a bit of background. I trained as a doctor at

the Royal Free Hospital in London. After qualifying, I pursued a career in journalism, and for the last 30 years I have been making science and health-related documentaries for BBC Television – first behind the camera, more recently as a presenter. I've reported on many of the great medical issues of the last three decades and interviewed numerous experts on a huge range of topics. This experience has given me a unique perspective. So I'm not exaggerating when I say that the recent rise in diabesity (diabetes plus obesity) is truly scary.

To be honest, for most of my career I was not particularly interested in nutrition. There was next to nothing about the effects of food on the body in my medical training, beyond the obvious, "eat less, do more exercise", which may be true but is completely unhelpful.

A decade ago, if you had asked me what I knew about diets, I would have told you, with great certainty, that the best way to lose weight was gradually, and with a low-fat diet. A pound or two a week was best, because if you went faster you would wreck your metabolism and end up yo-yo dieting. I occasionally tried following my own advice, lost a little weight, then put it straight back on. I didn't realise at the time just how bad my own advice was.

Then, three years ago, I went to see my doctor and had a routine blood test. A few days later she rang to say that not only was my cholesterol too high, but my blood sugar was in the diabetic range. Only just, but none-the-less, diabetic. Time to go on the tablets. I was shocked and wondered what to do. Because I knew, even then, that this is not a trivial disease.

I shouldn't have been surprised. Blood sugar problems are often inherited, and when my father died at the relatively early age of 74 he was suffering from a wide range of diseases, including type 2 diabetes, heart failure, prostate cancer and what I now suspect was early dementia.

Rather than start on a lifetime of medication I decided to make a documentary for the BBC in which I would seek out alternative ways to improve my health.

While making that documentary *Eat, Fast, Live Longer*, I came across the work of scientists like Professor Mark Mattson at the National Institute on Aging and Dr Krista Varady at the University of Illinois in Chicago who were researching something called "intermittent fasting".

Years of animal research and numerous human trials have shown the multiple benefits to be had from periodically reducing your calorie intake. These include not only weight loss but improvements in mood and memory.

So I went on what I called the 5:2 diet (eat normally five days a week and cut calories to around 600 on the other two days) and found it surprisingly manageable. I lost 20lb in 12 weeks and my blood sugar levels and cholesterol levels returned to normal. After making the documentary I wrote a book, with Mimi Spencer, called *The Fast Diet*, which included not only the science behind intermittent fasting but also a practical guide on how to do it (for more information visit thefastdiet.co.uk).

Our book was not, however, aimed at diabetics, and I wondered at the time if what had happened to me was unusual. So I decided to look more closely into the science linking calories, carbohydrates, obesity, insulin and diabetes. That quest has resulted in this book.

Why now?

Standard nutritional advice is under attack like never before. The age-old instruction to "eat low fat" has been seriously undermined by numerous studies which show that such a regime is rarely effective and people who go on it rarely stick to it.

The trouble is that when people cut out fat they get hungry, so they switch to eating cheap and sugary carbs, one of the main causes of the dietary disaster we face today.

And yet, despite everything, the standard advice has barely changed. For decades governments warned of the dangers of fat while ignoring the dangers of sugary carbs. Many of us know what our cholesterol levels are but few of us know what our blood sugar is doing, let alone our insulin levels. And we should be concerned, because blood sugar levels are rising at unprecedented rates.

There are now nearly four million diabetics in the UK and a recent shock finding[1] was that those with prediabetes (blood sugar levels that are abnormally high but not yet in the diabetic range) have more than tripled in the last 10 years, up from 11% to over 35%.

According to the CDC (Centers for Disease Control), things are worse in the US. There are at least 29 million people with diabetes and many don't know they have it.

The singer Patti LaBelle only discovered she was a type 2 diabetic when she passed out on stage. Her mother, also diabetic, had her legs amputated and her uncle went blind because of the disease.

The number with prediabetes is even greater. The CDC estimates that it affects 86 million Americans, with less than 1 in 10 being aware they are at risk.

Asians are particularly vulnerable: recent estimates suggest more than 100 million Chinese now have diabetes, while 500 million have prediabetes. Again, most are blissfully unaware.[2]

And prediabetes matters, not just because it normally leads to diabetes but also because it is closely linked to metabolic syndrome, sometimes called Syndrome X or insulin resistance syndrome.

You may or may not have heard of metabolic syndrome – 10 years ago I hadn't, but now it's incredibly common. And it is on the rise. Metabolic syndrome is also known as the "Deadly Quartet" because, as well as raised blood sugar, it includes hypertension, abdominal obesity and abnormal levels of cholesterol and fat in the blood.

Linking them all is the hormone insulin, which you'll be reading a lot more about in this book.

If you have prediabetes (and unless you've been tested you won't know), then there's roughly a 30% chance that you will go on to develop diabetes within five years.

The actor Tom Hanks was warned by his doctor that he was likely to become a diabetic well before he did, because of persistently high blood sugar levels. Hanks was not particularly overweight, but he was probably carrying too much weight for his particular genetic make-up. I'll be talking more about "personal fat thresholds" later.

Once you tip from prediabetes into diabetes you will be slapped on medication faster than you can say "Coca-Cola".

While I was researching this book, I received an email from the daughter of a diabetic. "My mum is embarrassed," she wrote. "She thinks it is her fault that she has developed type 2 diabetes. She has always been ashamed of being overweight and yet, despite her best efforts, has never been able to lose the weight. She has not even told my dad (who she lives with!) that she has diabetes, and she only told me because I saw her taking some pills and asked her what they were for."

Pills are the obvious answer. But they don't treat the underlying disease and there are question marks about their long-term effectiveness.

Anyway, I'm convinced that there are lots of people who, given the opportunity, would rather get healthy through lifestyle changes than resort to a lifetime on drugs. The tragedy is that they are rarely given the chance.

In this book I'm going to put the case for a different and surprising way to combat diabesity and rising blood sugar – and that is to go on a rapid weight loss diet.

But surely, I hear you say, that's crash dieting and crash dieting always fails? You end up putting back on all the weight you lost, and more. Well, no. Like anything, it depends on how it is done. Done badly, a very low-calorie diet will cause misery. Done properly, rapid weight loss is an extremely effective way to shed fat, combat blood sugar problems, reverse type 2 diabetes, perhaps even cure it.

I am going to take you through the science and demolish many common myths around dieting. And on the way you're going to have to embrace some radical ideas. I will introduce you to Professor Roy Taylor, the inspiration for this book. Professor Taylor is one of Europe's most respected diabetes researchers and he has shown, in several trials, that a very low-calorie diet can, in just a few weeks, do what was once seen as impossible – reverse type 2 diabetes. You will also meet the people who have used his approach to diet their way back to health:

- Carlos, a man on the brink of death, who now feels – and looks – 20 years younger.

- Lorna, who had no idea her blood sugar was out of control because she was a fit, healthy vegetarian.

- Geoff, who was about to have a foot

amputated, and who wants to save others from going down the same road.

- Cassie, a nurse who developed type 2 diabetes when she was just 24. Prescribed with insulin, she, like many others who start on medication, then put on lots of weight, so much so that she was recently offered weight loss surgery. By following the diet outlined in this book, she lost 20kg (44lb) in two months. She is no longer on drugs and has never felt better.

- And Dick, my friend who also lost 20kg in eight weeks and reversed his blood sugar problems while still enjoying his food and drink. A year later, he is in the best shape I've seen him in for a long time.

These people are not exceptional. Despite being told by their doctors, "It won't work and you'll never stick to it," hundreds of others have done the same.

After losing weight, the real challenge, of course, is to keep it off. I will give you clear guidance on the changes you'll need to make to ensure your weight remains steady.

So, do you want to lose weight, improve your health and get your blood sugar under control? Do you want to achieve this while eating tasty, wholesome food? Well, you're in the right place.

The Blood Sugar Diet

- A short, sharp and effective solution to blood sugar problems

- Based on scientific trials

- A clear, precise 8-week plan

- Inspiring stories of other people's success

- Advice on what to do after you've lost the weight

In the next few chapters I'm going to explain why blood sugar matters and what happens if you don't do something about it.

But first, I want to tell you about Jon.

"I've found a way to live and to eat."

Jon remembers the moment when he first heard he had type 2 diabetes. It was March 17, 2012. The graphic designer, then 48, a father of two teenage sons, was busy with work. His phone rang – it was his doctor's receptionist. "You need to come in straightaway. Do you feel OK?" she asked anxiously. "Have you got someone with you?"

"I think they were worried I was about to go

into a coma," Jon says. Like many people with this condition, he had no idea that he had a problem. Yet his recent test showed his blood sugar levels were more than three times over the limit.

People in Jon's age group are developing type 2 diabetes faster than ever before, and in greater numbers than adults over 65, the group that's traditionally been linked with blood sugar problems.

Jon was put on medication and sent off to talk to nutritionists and dieticians.

What followed was months of conflicting advice. One "expert" told him to eat a whole pineapple every day. Another recommended cereal every morning. No one suggested cutting back his calories, despite the fact that he weighed 21st.

When he heard about the Blood Sugar Diet he was immediately attracted.

It made sense. He liked the fact that it got quick results. He liked the simplicity.

He waited until the day after his 49th birthday party. He was hung over. Yet despite feeling terrible he was ready to begin a new way of eating which he now says has been "life-changing".

He lost 19lb (8.5kg) in the first week. I'll repeat that, shall I? 19lb – literally, the same weight as a car tyre. Much of that would have been water, but still, it was impressive.

He was staggered – and immediately motivated to keep going. For the first time he remembers being able to wear socks and not feel the elastic digging into his swollen ankles. He dropped a jean size in seven days. "It was such a spur," he says, looking back. "I could see straight away that this was going to work."

Jon is a warm, funny guy who likes to party. So he fell off the wagon. Repeatedly. "I didn't beat myself up," he says. "I'd just start up again the following day." (It's true that when he sent me his weekly food diaries there was more than the occasional glass of prosecco.)

"Once I got going I stopped thinking about it as a diet. I just decided that this was the way I was going to eat." He started walking more and getting around by bicycle, further burning up the fat stores.

In three months, he lost 50lb (22.5kg). Friends and family say he looks 20 years younger. He is no longer on his diabetes medication. His blood sugar results are normal. He uses words like "control", "habit" and "automatic".

"This feels entirely sustainable," he says. "I've found a way to live and to eat."

To eat – and to live. That's what this book is all about.

SECTION I

THE SCIENCE

Chapter one

THE OBESITY EPIDEMIC: WHY WE'RE IN THE STATE WE'RE IN

A very recent phenomenon

Jon had a serious weight problem, but so, increasingly, does the rest of the world. And this has not crept up on us gradually. People became a bit heavier in the postwar years, but obesity took off in a spectacular fashion at the beginning of the 1980s; in a single generation it swept the globe.

The fattest people on earth now live in places like Mexico, Egypt and Saudi Arabia. Countries like China and Vietnam, though still relatively lean, have seen the numbers of overweight adults triple in less than 40 years.

Amongst the rich, developed countries it is the Americans, British and Australians who currently lead the pack, with roughly two-thirds of the population overweight. Men and women in these countries have put on an average of 18lb, or 8kg (the equivalent of a medium-sized suitcase), in the last three decades, much of it round the gut.

Children are particularly at risk. The only type of diabetes that used to be seen in children was type 1, in which the immune system mistakenly attacks the cells responsible for blood sugar control. Now many more are coming into clinics with type 2, which is largely due to weight and lifestyle. A three-year-old girl in the US, weighing 77lb (35kg), was recently in the news as one of the youngest type 2 diabetics yet seen.

A poor diet affects not just this generation but the next. Overweight mothers are having ever larger babies, who in turn are programmed by the rich diet they get in the womb to becoming obese in later life.

Obesity spreads like a virus, with family and friends being a major influence on what and how much we eat and what we consider "normal". Being a bit on the chubby side is socially acceptable. There are size 20 models; muffin tops and double chins are out and proud. But, while celebrating curviness has been, in many ways, a desirable response to unrealistic skinny supermodels, it remains a sad fact that too much fat in the wrong places has serious consequences.

So what triggered this explosion?

The obvious answer is that we eat more. In the US, average calorie intake has increased by over 25% since the late 1970s, which would easily account for the average weight rise of Americans.

But in that same period consumption of saturated fats, like butter, actually fell. The really big surge, which began in 1980, was in carbohydrates, particularly refined grains, up by a whopping 20% in just 15 years.

A study in the *American Journal of Clinical Nutrition*,[3] which compared what Americans have been eating for the last few decades and rates of diabetes, could find no link between the disease and the amount of fat and protein being devoured. Instead, they blame the rise of diabesity on falling levels of fibre in the diet, combined with a dramatic rise in the consumption of refined carbs. And what almost everyone now acknowledges is that the rise in refined carbs came about as an unintended consequence of the war on fat.

The rise and rise of carbohydrates

In 1955 President Eisenhower had a heart attack that nearly killed him. At that time heart disease was rampant in the US and so the hugely influential American Heart Association decided, on the basis of what turned out to be rather flimsy evidence, to declare war on saturated fat. Out with steak, butter, full-fat milk and cheese. In with margarine, vegetable oils, bread, cereals, pasta, rice and potatoes.

The man who convinced the American Heart Association, and then the rest of the world, to pursue this path was a physiologist called Ancel Keys. In the 1950s he did a study which compared fat consumption and deaths from heart disease in men from six different countries.

He showed that men in the US, who got a lot of their calories from fat, were far more likely to die from heart disease than men in Japan, who ate little fat. The link seemed clear and compelling.

The fact that the Japanese also ate far less sugar and processed foods was discounted. The fact that some countries enjoy high rates of fat consumption and yet have low levels of heart disease, such as France, was dismissed as an anomaly.

The American Heart Association gave Keys their support, their blessing, and the anti-fat campaign began in earnest. It took a while to get going, but by the 1980s there had been a dramatic change in what people were eating all around the world. Huge numbers followed medical advice and switched from eating animal fats, like butter and milk, to eating margarine, low-fat products and vegetable oils.

The campaign against saturated fat was not just based on fear that it would clog up arteries. Eating fat, it was widely believed, *made you fat*. Ounce for ounce, fat contains more calories than either carbohydrates or protein. So the easiest way, it was thought, to lose weight was to cut down on it.

Low-fat diets were now created and endorsed enthusiastically by the medical profession. My father tried quite a few and lost weight on each. The trouble was he found them impossible to stick to. He was not alone. The success rate of low-fat diets, even ones that are closely supervised and where patients are highly motivated, has been poor.

A poignant example of this was the Look Ahead trial in 2001.[4] Sixteen medical centres in the US recruited more than 5000 overweight diabetics to take part in a randomised controlled trial. Half were offered standard care, the other half were put on a low-fat diet. The low-fat group got personal nutritionists, trainers and group support sessions – the best that money could buy.

The trial was due to run up until 2016 but was stopped after 10 years "for futility". The patients in the low-fat group had lost only a little more weight than the control group and there were no differences in rates of heart disease or strokes. The diabetic patients had managed to cut their fat consumption but that had not produced either the weight loss or the health benefits that were hoped for.

In the meantime, the campaign against fat was working very successfully, in the sense that the world now ate far more fat-free and fat-reduced "diet" products. But we didn't get slimmer; we became fatter.

Part of the problem was that food manufacturers, when they took out the fat, put in sugar to make their food more palatable. The low-fat Starbucks muffin, for instance (now discontinued, or at least I can no longer find it on the Starbucks website), used to contain 430 calories and the equivalent of 13 teaspoons of sugar.

People seemed to think that if a product said "fat-free" on the label, then it wouldn't make you fat. There were doctors telling the public that you can't get fat eating carbohydrates and one leading nutritional expert, Jean Mayer, said that prescribing a carbohydrate-restricted diet to the public was "the equivalent of mass murder".

I went to medical school in 1980, when the campaign against fat was in full flow. I gave up butter, cream and eggs. I rarely ate red meat and switched to skimmed milk and low-fat yoghurt, neither of which I enjoyed, but both of which I was sure were good for me.

Over the next few decades, despite much self-denial, I put on nearly 30lb or 14kg (I was a skinny little medical student) and my blood sugar soared. The high-carb, low-fat diet I was on wasn't making me healthier. It was doing the reverse.

Why?

Carbs and insulin

Well, the thing about carbs, particularly the easily digestible ones, such as sugar, but also breakfast cereals, pasta, bread and potatoes, is that they are easily broken down in the gut to release sugar into your system.

Your pancreas responds by producing insulin. One of insulin's main jobs is to bring high blood sugar levels down, and it does this by helping energy-hungry cells, such as those in your muscles, take up the sugar.

Unfortunately, an unhealthy diet and a low-activity

lifestyle can, over many years, lead to what's called "insulin resistance". Your body becomes less and less sensitive to insulin.

Your blood sugar levels creep up. And as they rise, your pancreas responds by pumping out more and more insulin. But it's like shouting at your kids. After a while they stop listening.

While your muscles are becoming insulin-resistant, however, insulin is still able to force surplus calories into your fat cells. The result is that, as your insulin levels rise, more and more energy is diverted into fat storage. The higher the insulin, the fatter you get.

And yet the more calories you tuck away as fat, the less you have to keep the rest of your body going.

It's a bit like buying fuel, but instead of putting it in the tank you put it in the boot of the car. The fuel gauge sinks, but your frantic attempts to top up fail because the fuel is going into the wrong place.

Similarly, your muscles, deprived of fuel, tell your brain to eat more. So you do. But because your high insulin levels are encouraging fat storage, you just get fatter while staying hungry.

Dr Robert Lustig, a renowned paediatric endocrinologist who has treated hundreds of overweight children, points out in his excellent book, *Fat Chance*, that understanding insulin is crucial to understanding obesity.

"There is no fat accumulation without the energy-storage hormone, insulin," he writes. "Insulin shunts sugar to fat. It makes your fat cells grow. The more insulin the more fat."

He argues that the main reason obesity levels have doubled over the last 30 years is that our bodies are producing far more insulin than ever before.

He blames the modern diet, rich in sugar and refined carbs, for pumping up our insulin levels, a claim supported by many other leading obesity experts, including Dr David Ludwig, a paediatrician from Harvard Medical School, and Dr Mark Friedman, head of the Nutrition Science Initiative in San Diego.

They recently wrote an opinion piece in the *New York Times* ("Always Hungry? Here's Why")[5] in which they point the finger firmly at refined carbs:

"The increasing amount and processing of carbohydrates in the American diet has increased insulin levels, put fat cells into storage overdrive and elicited obesity-promoting biological responses in a large number of people. High consumption of refined carbohydrates – chips, crackers, cakes, soft drinks, sugary breakfast cereals and even white rice and bread – has increased body weights throughout the population."

Dr Ludwig is worth listening to because he has run, for many years, one of the largest US clinics for overweight children at the Children's Hospital, Boston. He has seen, close up, how easily digestible carbs (those with a high glycaemic load, see page 93) have been a major driver of obesity.

In one study,[6] he took 12 overweight teenage boys and on separate days gave them three different breakfasts. One was instant oatmeal with milk and sugar. Another was traditional, unprocessed oats, "steel-cut", the sort your grandmother would recognise. The third breakfast was an omelette.

The worst breakfast was the instant oats. After eating it, the boys' blood sugar and insulin levels soared. This was followed a couple of hours later by a "crash" as blood sugar levels fell below where they had started. This crash was accompanied by a surge of the stress hormone, adrenaline. The boys felt tired, hungry and irritable. At lunch they each ate a whopping 620 calories more than those who had had the omelette.

From personal experience I know how this feels. If I eat toast or cereal I get hungry by mid-morning, while eating scrambled eggs, porridge or kippers for breakfast (even if these amount to the same number of calories) keeps me going well into the afternoon.

In another study,[7] Ludwig put 21 overweight young men on diets ranging from low-fat to low-carb. Despite eating exactly the same number of calories, those on the low-carb diet burnt 325 calories more per day than those on the low-fat diet. About as much energy as you would burn from an hour's jogging.

> *"By the time you are 50 you are going to have the body you deserve."*

This is what Bob Smietana used to eat:

Breakfast: cereal, muffins, coffee (several cups)
Lunch: hamburger, pizza, French fries, soda
Dinner: Two double cheeseburgers, big fries, soda, on the way home in the car.

This fatty, carb-driven diet is typical of what many people eat on a regular basis. It's not as though we don't know those big bags of chocolate are supposed to be for sharing. Or that that blueberry muffin won't count as one of our five a day. It's just that wodges of the white stuff – preferably sprinkled with sugar or salt – is so much easier to eat. Even if it does leave us feeling bloated one second... and starving the next.

Smietana is a journalist based in Chicago. He is an articulate, self-deprecating middle-class kinda guy, with two teenage children, a happy marriage and a successful career. During the time when he was on calorie overload, he had a lot on his plate (I'm talking metaphorically at this point). His work was stressful and he was worried about his wife who had been ill. Carby, convenient fast food was a comfort.

Except it wasn't, because he was bad-tempered

all the time, which wasn't like him. "I called myself 'Angry Bob,'" he says, looking back. "I was irritated constantly. Frustrated. Little things would make me go off on one. There was a tension in the air and it had grown over time." He wasn't sleeping well. He describes a mental fuzziness. Both are symptoms of blood sugar issues but people don't make the connection. "I was making mistakes at work. My thinking wasn't clear."

He was in his mid-forties. He weighed over 280lb (127kg) – he doesn't know exactly how much because after that point he refused to get on the scales. Smietana knew he didn't like what he could see in the mirror. Not long after this he was diagnosed with type 2 diabetes.

"The minute the diagnosis came, it was terrifying," recalls Smietana. He describes it now as a teachable moment. "I wanted to live to see my daughter get married. I wanted to be around to enjoy my grandchildren. But I knew I was walking slowly towards an early death.

"Changing your diet and your habits is such a huge thing," he says. "You think 'I can't do that.' You can't get started because you think it is too hard. The mountain is too big."

How did he do it? "Bit by bit. By moving in that direction and not thinking too much about how big this was. But it started with my own fear. The fear was a strength."

The first thing he did was get rid of the unhealthy carbohydrates. The second thing he did was eat more vegetables. His calorie intake plummeted. "The more I did it, the less I liked the wrong things." He lost 90lb (41kg).

The man who used to be a regular at his local McDonalds drive-in took up walking. "I will go for a walk now. Even if the world is on fire I will go for a walk because I know that is what I need to do." His next goal is to run a marathon.

"I am a great believer in habit," says Smietana. "Once you do something over and over again it becomes automatic and you stop thinking about it." He eats at the same time every day, he walks at the same time every day, he eats the same kind of things every day.

In retrospect he thinks we've become disconnected from our bodies. "We are on the phone or living virtual lives. We don't think about the physical side of life. We don't understand how our bodies work. Most people don't know what their pancreas does, what insulin is." Now, he can tell when his blood sugar is going out of balance – "I can tell immediately if I haven't exercised. My emotions are heightened – be it excitement or anger or angst."

It's easy to like Smietana. He is a thoughtful guy who quietly, with determination, dieted and walked his way back to health. He makes a vivid comparison with that other American obsession

– the automobile. "In my twenties I had a car and I knew how to mend it – how to change a tyre, for instance. Now I have no connection to it at all – we just replace our cars when they go wrong. We expect to be able to do the same with our bodies but we can't."

In 2015 his doctor – who was supportive throughout his diet – took him off his diabetes medication. His children also stopped calling him "Crazy Dad".

Blood sugar – the toxic timebomb

Although being obese, like Bob, can lead to type 2 diabetes, it's not inevitable. You can be overweight without being diabetic and diabetic without being overweight. In fact, being a skinny type 2 diabetic can be more dangerous than being a fat one. The real problem, as we'll see, is not how much fat you carry but where it gets deposited. If you lay down fat in the wrong places it can lead to high blood sugar, with all its potential complications, including the loss of a limb.

When I was a medical student I used to assist at operations. When I say "assist" all I really did was hold on to a retractor and laugh at the surgeon's jokes. I've watched plenty of successes and failures play out inside the operating theatre. But one of the saddest and most gruesome operations I attended was the removal of a patient's foot.

The patient was a man in his early fifties called Richard. I went to see him before his operation to take a medical history. I found him on the ward, lying in bed with his two feet sticking out of the end, "because I want to enjoy them for as long as I can". Richard was a successful lawyer, frightened but trying not to show it. He was a loving husband, a proud father. A couple of years earlier he'd found himself becoming increasingly tired and lethargic. He went to see his doctor, had tests, and discovered he was a type 2 diabetic.

Richard started taking tablets but soon progressed to insulin injections. He received no dietary advice, apart from being told to eat low-fat food and fill his plate with plenty of potatoes and pasta. He put on more and more weight.

Then one day he knocked the side of his foot against a chair. He developed a little blister. It got bigger. Then it got infected. It was downhill from there. "It was all so quick," I remember him saying. "I had no idea that it would get so bad so fast."

His surgeon attempted to repair what was now a gaping ulcer on his foot with a skin graft taken from elsewhere on his body, but it failed. Richard was advised that he would have to have his foot removed.

He told me he was in shock when he heard the news; terrified, didn't know what to say. He went home and told his wife. She broke down and cried.

A day after first meeting Richard I went to the operating theatre and watched the surgeon remove his foot, which was then carried away to be disposed of. He spent months in hospital recovering, and I never saw him again.

What raised blood sugar does to your body

Your blood vessels

The problem for Richard was that the raised sugar in his blood had stuck to proteins in the walls of his blood vessels, making them stiffer and less flexible. This, in time, had led to the build-up of scar tissue – plaque – inside his blood vessels. It had also damaged his nerves, so he could no longer feel pain when he bashed his leg.

If you'd looked inside Richard's eyes or the arteries supplying blood to his heart, you would have seen further damage. Diabetes is a major cause of blindness and more than doubles your risk of having a heart attack or stroke. It is also a leading cause of impotence.

And you don't have to have blood sugars in the diabetic range for damage to occur. In a big Australian study[8] in which they followed more than 10,000 men and women for a number of years, they found that, though being diabetic more than doubled your risk of dying, simply having blood sugar levels in the "impaired fasting glucose" range increased your risk of premature death by over 60%.

Your brain

My father started becoming confused towards the end of his life. He found it increasingly hard to remember names and was constantly forgetting conversations we'd had only a few hours before. He was convinced he was rich (which he wasn't) and began to give away money to strangers with hard-luck stories that he met in bars and restaurants. I suspect he was showing early signs of dementia, which may well have been linked to his diabetes.

We've known for many years that diabetics have an increased risk of becoming demented (partly because of blood supply problems), but it's only recently that we've seen just how big the risk really is. In a recent study in Japan[9] in which they followed more than 1000 men and women for 15 years, they found that being diabetic doubled your risk of dementia.

Dr Suzanne De La Monte, a neuropathologist at Brown University, says that diabetes doesn't inevitably lead to dementia, but it's certainly an important factor. "Alzheimer's disease occurs in people without diabetes, and vice versa," she says. "But I think type 2 diabetes is pushing up rates of Alzheimer's disease like crazy."

Your looks

Last, and by no means least, raised blood sugar will make you look older by attacking the collagen and elastin molecules in your skin; this in turn makes your face saggy, baggy and wrinkled.

In a striking demonstration of this, researchers from Leiden University in the Netherlands[10] measured the blood sugar of over 600 volunteers. They then asked a group of independent assessors to try and guess their age.

People with low blood sugar were perceived to be significantly younger than their real age, while the reverse was true of the wrinklies with high blood sugar. The researchers estimate that every additional mmol/l increase in blood sugar adds five months to your "perceived age".

Diabetes – the physical costs

Hypertension: 70% of diabetics also require medication for blood pressure.

Cholesterol: 65% of diabetics require medication to reduce their cholesterol.

Heart attacks: Diabetics, even when on full medication, are twice as likely to be hospitalised, crippled or die from a heart attack.

Strokes: Diabetics are 1.5 times more likely to suffer a debilitating stroke.

Blindness and Eye Problems: Diabetes is the number one cause of preventable blindness in the developed world.

Impotence: Diabetes is also the number one cause of impotence.

Dementia: Having diabetes doubles your risk of dementia.

Kidney disease: Diabetes is the cause of kidney failure in half of all new cases; most people on dialysis are diabetics.

Amputations: There are over 7000 diabetes-related amputations done every year in the UK and over 73,000 in the US.

Chapter two

HOW DO YOU SOLVE A PROBLEM LIKE DIABETES?

So if you've got type 2 diabetes or prediabetes, can you reverse it, possibly cure yourself?

This is a question that Roy Taylor answers with an empathic "Yes". He is Professor of Medicine and Metabolism at Newcastle University, where he also runs the Diabetes Research Group. He is slim and active, and has a dry sense of humour.

While his supporters say his very low-calorie diet has turned their lives around, he's met a lot of opposition. The first time he tried to publish a paper about his findings it was turned down. The editors didn't believe the results.

"People don't think it is real," says Professor Taylor. "Yes, you might be able to do it in a freak study but it is not relevant. What you were told as a medical student and what you have been told your entire medical career is that people with type 2 diabetes get steadily worse and eventually end up on insulin. There are plenty of articles in the medical press which state firmly that the first thing someone ought to do when they are told they have type 2 is accept the diagnosis. And then I come along and tell them that might not be true."

Recently one of his high-profile critics approached him after a lecture. "I was wrong," he told him. "You were right." If Professor Taylor was the type to punch the air he might have done so.

What makes resistance to Professor Taylor's research so surprising is that for many years there has been clear evidence that type 2 can be reversed through dramatic weight loss – most notably through bariatric (weight loss) surgery.

Professor Taylor came across the link between bariatric surgery and diabetes in the 1980s, when he visited Greenville, North Carolina, a city with very high rates of obesity. Professor Taylor said people used to stare when he walked down the street. "I don't think they were used to seeing such a thin guy."

One of the surgeons based in Greenville was Walter Pories. He not only operated on obese patients, but also did long-term follow-up studies to find out what happened to them afterwards.

One study, with the lengthy title "Who would have thought it? An operation proves to be the most effective therapy for adult-onset diabetes mellitus",[11] followed 608 seriously obese patients for 14 years. Not everyone improved, but in most cases the weight loss was spectacular. By the end of year one the patients had, on average lost a third of their total body weight (100lb or 45kg), a weight loss that they maintained till the end of the study, 14 years later. Along with a fall in weight there were impressive falls in blood pressure, improvements in sleep and a big drop in their risk of dying from heart disease.

Perhaps the most impressive changes, however, were in those who had blood sugar problems: of the 608 patients in the study, 161 had type 2 diabetes and 150 had impaired glucose tolerance (prediabetes).

For most of these patients there was a dramatic fall in blood sugar levels after surgery. As the researchers observed, "The diabetes cleared rapidly, generally in a matter of days, to the degree that most diabetic bariatric surgical patients were discharged without any anti-diabetic medications."

One patient, on huge doses of insulin, was able to stop her insulin within a week of surgery and within three months her blood sugars had returned to normal. Even more impressively, 14 years later, she, like 83% of the former diabetics, was still "normal".

The ones who didn't respond as well were those who had been diabetic for many years before the surgery.

Those who were prediabetic – with blood sugar high but not yet in the danger zone – had the best results of all. In 99% of them blood sugar levels went back to normal and stayed there.

Surgery, it ought to be said, is not an easy option. Although death rates are low, patients sometimes have to be readmitted to hospital to be treated for infections or because their wounds break down. The operation can also lead to "dumping syndrome" after eating, which is as unpleasant as it sounds. Your heart rate soars, you have butterflies in your stomach and profuse diarrhoea.

The researchers had noticed that surgery produced changes in gut hormones, the hormones that control appetite. So they assumed the dramatic improvements in blood sugar had to be something to do with the way the surgery itself had changed the hormones.

Professor Taylor, however, was not convinced. "I know about gut hormones; they are very important, but they have limited effect on metabolic changes. I knew right away this claim had to be wrong. But it became the established belief, the belief throughout the scientific world: a change in gut hormones explains why blood sugars return to normal after surgery."

He thought there was a completely different explanation, one that could explain why many overweight people don't get diabetes, while many slim people do.

The worst places to pile on the fat – it's not where you think

Insulin decides *whether* you get fat, but it is an enzyme called lipoprotein lipase (LPL) that decides *where* you get fat.

We don't become fat all over (we don't have fat foreheads); we lay it down in certain places. And whether it is around your middle, your thighs, your bottom or your hips, depends largely on LPL. Once activated, this enzyme will, with the help of insulin, suck the fat out of your blood and stick it in storage.

Men tend to have more LPL in the fat cells of their bellies, which is why we put on fat around our waists. Women, on the other hand, are more likely to have active LPL in the fat cells of the hips and the bottom, which is why it piles on there.

The good news is that LPL is also found in muscles. If you activate the LPL in your muscles by exercising, then surplus calories running round your system are more likely to be dumped in them to be burnt as energy, instead of stored as fat.

A few years ago, while making a documentary, *The Truth About Exercise*, I took part in an experiment at Glasgow University to demonstrate the difference even a modest amount of exercise can make.

The experiment consisted of eating a large, greasy breakfast full of fried foods, like bacon, eggs and haggis. An hour later I had some blood taken by Dr Jason Gill. He put it into a sophisticated centrifuge to separate the red cells from the plasma.

When this was done he showed me, floating on top of my plasma, a murky layer of fat. This was the fat that I had eaten at breakfast and which was now travelling around my arteries.

He then asked me to go for a brisk one-hour walk, which I did. The following morning we repeated the process: I ate a greasy breakfast, after which my blood was taken and spun down.

This time, however, the layer of fat on top of my plasma was much thinner. The walk I had done the previous afternoon had switched on genes in my leg muscles, activating the LPL enzymes in them, which had then sucked much of the fat out of my blood.

Unfortunately, most of us don't go for long, vigorous walks after a meal or indeed at any other time. A far more likely fate for the calories from a slap-up meal is that the insulin in your blood will direct them into fat cells. Some will become subcutaneous fat, which gathers on your bottom, thighs and arms. That is relatively harmless. But the rest will become visceral fat, which is a hidden fat that wraps itself around your heart, liver and gut. Because this fat lies inside the body, rather than on the surface where you can see it, you can appear to be relatively slim.

People like that are known in the trade as TOFIs, Thin on the Outside, Fat Inside.

I used to be one of them.

Visceral or internal fat is particularly dangerous because it invades organs, like your liver and pancreas.

Fatty liver and pancreas – the heart of the problem

We don't think of our livers as being "fatty", but the liver is actually one of the first places that fat gets stored. It is like your current account at the bank: a quick and easy place to put away spare cash. But it is an account, as Professor Taylor puts it, "with a punishingly high interest rate", because it can lead to all sorts of problems – not just abnormal blood sugar levels but also non-alcoholic fatty liver disease (NAFLD). Thirty per cent of Europeans and Americans have NAFLD, which can lead to cirrhosis and liver failure. It is the commonest cause of liver disease in the West.

Professor Taylor's research suggests that it is the build-up of fat inside the liver and pancreas that causes all the trouble. These two organs are responsible for controlling our insulin and blood sugar levels. As they get clogged up with fat they stop communicating with each other. Eventually your body stops producing insulin and you become a type 2 diabetic.

Professor Taylor also argues that we have our own "personal fat threshold" (PFT), a tipping point, which is partly down to genetics. Your tipping point decides how much fat you can accumulate before it starts to overflow into your liver and pancreas, leading to type 2.[12]

In some people the PFT seems to be set high, in others surprisingly low.

The good news is that whatever your PFT may be, if

you drain the fat out of your liver and pancreas (and the diet in this book helps you do just that), then you can reverse your diabetes and restore your blood sugars to normal. The bad news is that, if you don't sort it out, you will not only get the complications of diabetes but may also permanently damage your liver.

> *"People would tell me: 'Lorna, you have nothing to worry about. You are thin.'"*

Lorna Norman's doctor was shocked when a blood test revealed that Lorna had blood sugar problems. "You'll be as staggered as I am."

Lorna is vegetarian and had always eaten healthily. She exercised her dogs every day. She swam regularly. She had never had a health scare before. Apart from tiredness – which was what had prompted her to go to her doctor in the first place – she had no symptoms.

Her doctor sent her to see a nurse, who told her not to worry, and to carry on as normal. "In hindsight," says Lorna, "that was the last thing I needed to do." (Common mistake number 1.)

"People would tell me: Lorna, you have nothing to worry about. You are thin. You look fine." (Common mistake number 2.)

She carried on eating plenty of carbohydrates.

Pasta. Bread. Baked potatoes. (Common mistake number 3.) "Now I know that was completely the wrong thing to eat, but that was what the experts were telling me to do." And for several years her results hovered around the borderline mark.

But then they gradually began to creep up, like a patch of damp on a wall. When she stepped on the scales she was 133lb (60kg) – not overweight for her height, 5ft 4in. But – and this is key – her excess weight had a tendency to sit around her middle.

On her next visit to the doctor her blood sugar had gone up again. It was the news she had dreaded. She was diabetic and her doctor told her she needed to start on medication immediately. (Common mistake number 4.)

When Lorna told her doctor about Roy Taylor's research that suggested that a very low-calorie diet could take her blood sugar levels back down to normal, he was sceptical. "He told me, 'You are not overweight and your BMI [Body Mass Index] is fine. You really shouldn't be on this kind of diet.' He thought it was nonsense." (Common mistake number 5.)

She decided to go ahead. "I just thought I am going to have a stab at anything that stops me from going on medication." There's a pause. "My daughter might say I am a control freak."

It took four weeks for her BMI to go down to

19. She was strict. She made sure she was getting enough of the right nutrients. She drank three litres of water a day. It wasn't all plain sailing. Her results improved but there were points when her blood sugar levels started going up again. "I thought I must be one of those people for whom it didn't work." (Common mistake number 6.)

She kept going – and stopped testing herself so often, which helped her not to worry so much. She also took up yoga and meditation ("I put the laundry on and meditate until the beep goes"). Her stress levels fell and brought down the blood-sugar-bamboozling hormone, cortisol.

Amazingly she managed to do all this and still cater for three other adults in the house. She even continued to do all the cooking. "I would do their meals and then sit down to whatever little plate of food that I was having."

She was 8st 7lb (54kg) at her lightest. "Lots of people commented on how thin I looked but frankly I didn't care. People are more likely to tell you how you look than they are to congratulate you for not having a life-threatening illness any longer. It's very peculiar."

After two months she was diabetes-free. The reduction in her waist measurement from 34 to 30in was probably the crucial factor in this.

What's wrong with just taking pills?

As we all know, losing weight and keeping it off requires effort. So if your doctor tells you, "Yes, you have type 2 diabetes, but it's easily treatable with tablets," then you are probably going to take the easy way out.

But diabetes is rarely that simple. Even if you are treated with medication, being a diabetic can take 10 years off your life.

It will also cost you, or whoever has to cover your medical expenses, a great deal of money. It's not just the cost of the drugs, the cost of treating the complications and the time off work. Having a diagnosis of type 2 diabetes will also make getting life insurance and health insurance harder and more expensive. Even travel insurance will have an added premium, because of the increased risks.

In the UK it's estimated that type 2 diabetes costs the country at least £20 billion a year. In the US it's more like $245 billion.

The bestselling anti-diabetes drug on the market at the moment is metformin, with sales of nearly $2 billion a year. It has been around for so long and used on so many people that you would imagine it must be really effective. Yet a recent paper[13] that looked at the results of 13 randomized controlled trials involving more than 13,000 patients could find little compelling evidence that taking the drug reduces heart attacks or leg amputations or improves life expectancy.

At least metformin can lead to modest weight reduction (possibly because common side effects include nausea), but it is normally only the first step on a road that leads to more powerful and expensive anti-diabetes drugs. And most of these other drugs, including insulin, promote hunger, which makes patients fatter. As one expert told me, "The more aggressively we treat them, the fatter they get."

The current situation with diabetes reminds me, in some ways, of the first television documentary I ever made, back in the early 1990s. It was called *Ulcer Wars* and it was about a young Australian doctor called Barry Marshall.

At that time stomach ulcers were a very common and painful condition caused, as everyone knew, by the production of too much acid in the stomach.

It was widely believed that the increased acid was the result of stress and a poor lifestyle. You had brought this condition on yourself by living badly.

Fortunately the wonderful pharmaceutical companies had developed drugs which could reduce the symptoms by reducing the acid levels in your stomach. But because this was an incurable disease you had to go on taking expensive drugs for the rest of your life or the ulcer would return.

Dr Marshall, however, was not convinced by this explanation. He believed that stomach ulcers were actually caused by previously unknown bacteria, *Helicobacter pylori*, which he and a colleague, Robin Warren, had discovered in the stomachs they had had to remove from unfortunate patients whose ulcers had burst.

They tried, and failed, to infect animals in the lab with *Helicobacter*, so in the end Marshall decided to infect himself. He didn't tell his wife because, as he candidly told me, "she would have tried to stop me".

Before doing anything he persuaded a colleague to push an endoscopic tube down his throat and take a good look at his stomach. It was completely normal.

Then he asked a technician to brew up a beaker of bacteria (grown from an infected patient's stomach) and swallowed it in one go. Not the sort of thing you would want to sip.

A few days later he became ill and vomited. He was thrilled.

He had himself endoscoped again, and this time the surgeon saw patches of inflammation. He took samples of Marshall's stomach, and when they looked down the microscope they saw bacteria swarming through the tissue.

Marshall's wife now insisted that he stop the experiment, so he took a cocktail of antibiotics and a medicine called Pepto-Bismol (which is mildly toxic to bacteria); a few days later his symptoms improved.

By the time I made my documentary with Barry Marshall he, and others, had treated a lot of patients and shown that you could not only cure most stomach ulcers with antibiotics but also reduce their chance of developing stomach cancer.

Yet few doctors were listening and the only response to my film from the medical profession was a review in the *British Medical Journal* that described it as "one-sided and tendentious". Which is medical speak for "garbage".

Within a few years, however, the evidence was so overwhelming and patient demand so great that use of antibiotic triple therapy became widespread. In 2000 Barry Marshall and Robin Warren won the Nobel Prize for Medicine.

Like stomach ulcers, you can certainly control diabetes with drugs. But wouldn't it be far better to treat the underlying cause? If you had an infection wouldn't you want to get rid of it, before it progresses, rather than merely treat the symptoms?

"Doctors will argue that they are too busy to monitor weight loss. But it could save them a hell of a lot of time in the long term if they did."

It took Colin Beattie four months to wear down his doctor. Luckily he is a politician – he's a member of the Scottish Parliament – so he knows how to make an argument. And repeat it. Again and again.

The 63-year-old had been diagnosed with type 2 diabetes four years before and to begin with he barely gave the diagnosis a second thought. He was told to take one metformin tablet in the morning and another in the evening. Two years later – because his blood sugar levels were still rising – his dose needed to be doubled. So now he was on four tablets a day. The next thing he knew he was being put on statins. Towards the end of 2013, on his next visit to the doctor, he was informed that his blood pressure was too high – another pill was prescribed, this time to dilate the blood supply to his kidneys.

It was at this point that Colin began to seriously wonder about the ever-mounting pile of pills. "I started thinking – hang on. Is this what life is going to be like? More and more tablets?"

Colin did some research. He discovered Professor Taylor's work on very low-calorie diets and the potential to reverse type 2 diabetes. His doctor wasn't keen. "He was clearly worried he would have a flood of people coming into the surgery asking for help on the diet and that the surgery wouldn't be able to cope," he says.

Until then the dietary advice Colin had been given was basic. Eat more fruit and vegetables, avoid fatty food. "It seemed like an ordinary well-intentioned admonition to eat better." Predictably Colin pretty much ignored the advice (well, you would, wouldn't you, if your doctor seemed to think you should keep on taking the tablets and not worry?). "I tended to eat what I could, when I could. Fish and chips, steak pie, snacks between meals… A typical Scotsman's diet," he explains.

Gradually his doctor tired of the former invest-ment banker sitting opposite him, brandishing bundles of facts and figures about why a crash diet could work. Most reluctantly, he gave Colin the go-ahead and agreed to monitor his progress. This included a blood test at the beginning, looking at a weekly email from Colin stating his weight and blood pressure, and letting him know when he could begin to cut back on his medication. Colin was not, after all, as high-maintenance as his doctor feared.

What Colin did – and I think this was key to his success – was approach the diet as though it were a pharmaceutical regime. This was *prescrip-tion weight loss*. Because his day-to-day life is so high pressured and variable, he decided to use diet products rather than eat "real" food. Each meal break was 200 calories – so a typical day was a sachet of porridge for breakfast, soup for lunch, a diet bar for dinner, plus a plate of steamed vegeta-bles. That added up to 800 calories.

"I did two things that I think helped," he says now. "I made sure everyone knew I was going to do it – including the press. That helped keep the pressure on me. And I was absolutely determined that I wasn't going to break the diet. I knew if I did it would be easier to break it the next time and the next time. I absolutely stuck to it until the last day." (When he went out and ate a steak pie. Least said about that the better, but it goes to show he's human.)

Over eight weeks he lost 44lb (20kg). His waist shrank from 40 to 34in. By the end he was free of his medication.

Colin – despite the occasional steak pie – has managed to keep the weight off. When it creeps up a pound or two he cuts back. He is on a mission now to spread the word about low-calorie diets. He has been amazed by how many people have told him that they, too, are type 2 and shocked by how little support they get. "Doctors will argue that they are busy and don't have the time to monitor weight loss. But it could save them a hell of a lot of time in the long term if they did deal with it."

There are 236,000 type 2 diabetics in Scotland (not counting the people who don't know they've got it). Among those newly diagnosed last year were five children under four years old.

The Newcastle study

Professor Taylor was pretty sure that if he could get a diabetic patient to lose enough weight the fat would drain out of their pancreas and liver and their diabetes would be reversed. But because so many other doctors were sceptical, he knew he was going to have to put together a very convincing case.

First he needed to be able to measure what was actually happening to the levels of liver and pancreatic fat in his patients. Just sticking needles in was never an option.

Kieran Hollingsworth, a physicist in his department, had already adapted their MRI machines to measure liver fat. When Professor Taylor asked him, "Can you do this in the pancreas?" he paused, stared up at the ceiling for a moment before saying, "Yes."

Next he needed money to do a trial. "I was very fortunate," he said, "to get money from the charity Diabetes UK. They thought it was extremely unlikely to work, but one particular person thought it sounded interesting and managed to persuade the rest of the committee. It wasn't much. Enough for a small one-year study."

With the funding in place they recruited 14 patients.[14] Three of the volunteers dropped out early, for a variety of reasons, leaving 11 to soldier on.

These 11 were taken off their normal diabetes drugs and put on a strict regime of 800 calories a day, which consisted of liquid diet drinks and non-starchy vegetables.

In the first week they lost an average of 3.9kg (8lb) and most reported finding the diet surprisingly easy. "Much to my astonishment the hunger seems to disappear in 48 hours," Professor Taylor told me.

As the fat clogging up their livers melted away, their

symptoms improved. "The liver seemed to be fine after seven days and got better as time went by. The pancreas was slower to respond. It was a little better after seven days and then steadily improved over the next eight weeks – and that was the magic thing."

The volunteers stuck to the 800-calorie regime and in just eight weeks – a remarkably short time – lost an average of 15kg (33lb). They also lost nearly 5in round the waist. By the end their blood sugar levels were all back in the non-diabetic range.

Professor Taylor was astonished. "It was electrifying. Amazingly more definitive than I ever dreamt it would be."

Further studies

Alan, 56 and married with four sons, was part of that study. He was 97kg (213lb) when he was diagnosed with diabetes and essentially told, "You've got it, deal with it." When he heard that Professor Taylor was looking for volunteers he leapt at the chance. His own doctor was less enthusiastic. "Don't feel bad when you fail."

But Alan didn't fail. "I never felt that I was flagging or wanted to give up. I felt like a pioneer, that what I was doing was important."

In eight weeks Alan lost 13kg (29lb), almost 14% of his starting weight. Three years later he has kept most of that weight off and his blood sugar measurements remain in the healthy range.

"I'm no angel. I still have takeaways, wine, cheese, beer. I have a special black shirt that used to fit like cling film. I put it on every so often to see if it still fits. As long as it fits I'm doing fine."

Alan, like the other volunteers, had been recently diagnosed. Would it work with people who had been diabetic for longer?

In a follow-up study published in 2015,[15] Professor Taylor's team tested the diet on 29 people with type 2 diabetes, some of whom had been diabetic for more than eight years and some who had been diabetic for a while, but less than four years.

Again they found that people were surprisingly good at sticking to the diet and they got great results. In this trial 87% of the shorter-duration group and 50% of the long-duration group managed to get their fasting blood sugars back to normal without medication.

So does Professor Taylor have any concerns about people doing it outside a proper clinical setting?

"None," he replied, "but with two specific reservations, both of those related to drugs. If you are on anti-hypertensives, then you should discuss with your doctors either cutting down or stopping them before you start dieting. Your blood pressure is going to drop and it could go too low if drugs are continued. Similarly there are some glucose-lowering drugs, ones that begin with the letter G, like glibenclamide and gliclazide, which may have to be stopped because they can push your blood glucose abnormally low."

What would he say to those who worry about the potential dangers of going on a low-calorie diet for two months?

"The anxieties about fasting have been grossly exaggerated and it partly relates to poor-quality 400-calorie diets that were used long ago in the US for very long periods of time. With a balanced 800 calories for eight weeks I have absolutely no qualms at all, though ideally people should discuss their plans with their doctor or diabetes team to get personal medical advice."

So what does he think about doing it with real food rather than diet shakes?

"I'd rather people did. When the diet was first talked about publicly, 77 individuals did it off their own bat and half of them did it by eating real food. They lost the same amount of weight as we had achieved under controlled conditions in our studies. It can be done."

Professor Taylor's team have shown it is possible to reverse type 2 diabetes in motivated people. The really important thing now is to test this idea on a larger scale, find out who it's most suitable for and also, crucially, see what happens in the long term.

He and colleagues, including Mike Lean, Professor of Human Nutrition at Glasgow University, are currently involved in a much bigger study. Patients volunteering for DiRECT (Diabetes Remission Clinical Trial) are randomly allocated to either the current best-available type 2 diabetes care or the 800-calorie-a-day diet. The trial will run for five years and involve over 30 doctors' practices across the UK.

In the meantime, many individuals have been taking matters into their own hands.

"I was ready to die and suddenly I hear about a cure for this disease!"

Carlos Cervantes should be dead. There is no question in his mind about it. Indeed, just before the 55-year-old American discovered Professor Taylor's work – totally by chance, I'll tell you how in a second – he had concluded that his time was up. "I had decided that this was a good summer to die," he tells me. "It wasn't a low point. It was a realistic assessment of my situation."

This is what Carlos was up against: at his heaviest he weighed 305lb (138kg), his waist measured 56in, his toes were beginning to go black, he had a fungal infection in his ear and his doctor had warned him that an out-of-control foot ulcer meant he was looking at amputation. There were crutches beside the bed in his remote house on the slopes of Mount St Helens volcano in Washington State.

Insulin injections were no longer working. When he tested his blood sugar the machine could not process the reading. Again and again he tried. It turned out it was so high the figures were off the scale.

There are lots of reasons why this softly spoken man was in a fog of despair. Here are a few of them:

1. *His doctor had given up on him.* "It was very traumatic," he recalls. "I wasn't getting any help and I didn't know what was wrong with me. I was as sick as sick can be." His nickname for metformin was "MakeFatMan" because for him a side effect was even more weight gain. Carlos has a dark sense of humour.

2. *He had raging type 2 diabetes.* When fungus starts living off the sugar in your blood you're not talking borderline symptoms. According to every medical professional he spoke to, type 2 diabetes is a progressive illness and Carlos seemed to be in the final stages of it.

3. *He had followed lots of diets in the past. None of them worked.* Following the death of his mother from cancer when he was five, Carlos used food to compensate for the emotional loss. He was nine when, overweight and miserable, he began his first attempt at weight loss – the Atkins Diet. "That

didn't work for me," he laughs now. "Nothing ever really worked. I would lose weight and then it would all come back." He had a weakness for chocolate brownies. And then some.

4. *He was extremely stressed*. He was squeezed emotionally dry by major bereavements, a promising real estate business had been devastated by the credit crunch, and he was beset by financial worries.

And then, one day, he heard about the Newcastle Diet totally by chance. On Al Jazeera news. A two-minute news item. "I was ready to die and suddenly I hear about a cure for this disease!" What was that like?

"I think I busted a hole in the roof!" he replies. "I couldn't believe what I had heard." Carlos began doing his own research online and found an email address for Professor Taylor. He says, "I knew my doctor would tell me that it would not work. I decided to take matters into my own hands."

Carlos couldn't bear the shakes that were recommended so mostly he ate real food – just different from what he had been eating and a lot less of it. Vegetables, fruit, lean chicken, salad. Everything was carefully weighed out every day – if he had cheese, he would measure out a sliver. On the 10th day his blood sugar dropped for the first time. After

64 days he had lost 67lb (30kg) – the equivalent of an adult red setter dog. When he reached his target of 173lb (78kg), his diabetes had disappeared. "It cured me beyond my expectations," he says. "I would even call it a superhuman cure."

Since then he has changed the way he eats – most of the time.

He estimates he eats 95% healthy food, 5% junk. "At the centre of my plate is a pile of fresh, steamed vegetables, and around that is healthy grains. By the side is a piece of fish or chicken." He still occasionally eats chocolate cake or ice cream or tortilla chips but he says it does not affect him in the way it used to. "As a diabetic I couldn't eat any of those things. The diet cleaned out my liver and pancreas. It's not so easy for me to gain weight any more. I can get real skinny quickly. It's as though my body is working metabolically like a young man's again."

His trouser size is now 32in. "I like the person I see in the mirror now," he says. "Although sometimes it is hard to recognise myself. I had been morbidly obese my entire adult life."

He is a diabetes buddy at a nearby support group for people with issues around food. He begins our conversation with the words: "I will go to any lengths to bring the message of hope and recovery to any diabetic out there." Make no mistake about it – he is deadly serious.

Chapter three

ARE YOU AT RISK OF TYPE 2 DIABETES?

There is a close, but not inevitable link, between weight and the risk of developing blood sugar problems. It also depends on your age, gender and ethnicity.

If you are of white European descent you are more than twice as likely to develop type 2 diabetes if you have a Body Mass Index (BMI) over 30kg/m2 than if your BMI is less than 25kg/m2.

Because men have a greater tendency to put on weight around the gut, they develop type 2 diabetes at lower levels of BMI.

If you are of South Asian, Chinese, African-Caribbean or black African descent, then you are at increased risk. You will get diabetes at a lower BMI, earlier in life and go from being prediabetic to diabetic twice as quickly.

It's one reason why in countries like Vietnam, which have adopted a Western lifestyle, they are now amputating more limbs – due to the complications of diabetes – than at the height of the Vietnam War.

A condition that used to occur mainly in older people is skewing younger. It is far more serious if you get it in your thirties or forties than later in life. As one expert told me, "A 45-year-old man who gets it is likely to have his first major complication just 13 years later. People talk in terms of reduced life expectancy, but if you are a 45-year-old and you know that you might have to stop work early and be unable to support your family, that's scary."

Are you at risk of type 2 diabetes?

1. Do you have a diabetic parent, brother or sister?

    1 point

2. Are you being treated for hypertension?   1 point

3. Are you from a non-white ethnic background?

    1 point

4. Are you aged 50 to 59?   1 point

5. Are you over 60?   2 points

6. Is your waist over 35 but less than 42 inches?   1 point

7. Is your waist over 42 inches? (Measure your waist around the belly button, not your trouser size)   2 points

8. Is your Body Mass Index 25-30?   1 point

9. Is your BMI 31-35?   2 points

10. Is your BMI over 35?   3 points
    (To get your BMI score go to a website such as www.nhs.
    uk/tools/pages/healthyweightcalculator.aspx, which will
    calculate it for you.)

Add up your total score:

Less than 3 points: You have a low risk of becoming type 2 diabetic in
    the next 10 years.
3-5 points: You have a moderate risk of becoming diabetic and as
    you get older this risk will increase. Check your blood sugars and
    consider making life style changes so you can reduce your risk.
Over 5 points: You are at high risk of becoming diabetic. You should
    definitely have your blood sugars tested and aim for life style
    changes, such as significant weight loss and increased activity.

"I have been given another chance at life."
_____

Cassie was just 24 and pregnant when she was
started on diabetes medication. She had developed what's called "gestational diabetes", when
she was carrying her daughter, Grace.

Gestational diabetes is common – around 18%
of pregnant women get it. No one knows why, but
one theory is that hormones produced during pregnancy can block insulin receptors, making blood

sugar levels rise. It normally disappears after you've given birth.

Cassie's levels were so high that they put her on insulin. She hoped things would get better after her daughter was born. But they didn't.

Like many people who have a complex relationship with food, Cassie is insightful about what happened next. "I got into this cycle of guilt. Feeling guilty that I was a diabetic with a young child. Guilty about what I ate. One fuelled the other. In the end it seemed pointless trying to do anything about it – and then I ate more."

She was training to be a nurse. At work she would see people with type 2 diabetes and all the complications that the illness brings.

She was told to hold back on fatty foods, so she stocked up on carbs. Breakfast was crumpets, cereal, toast. Lunch would be sandwiches. Dinner, more often than not, was a takeaway. She would eat in secret as she was constantly hungry, perhaps because of all the insulin she was injecting. Over the next four years she put on a lot of weight.

When Cassie sent me an email she was so desperate to change that she was considering weight loss surgery. She had tried every diet going – among them Weight Watchers and Slimming World – and nothing had worked.

I wanted to help but she was on such high doses of insulin that I was worried what might happen. So

I passed her details on to my wife, Clare, who's a GP and sees a lot of diabetics.

Clare had a chat with Cassie and discovered that she has a supportive diabetic consultant. Importantly, she also knew exactly how to adjust her insulin to avoid "hypos" (when the blood sugar drops dangerously low due to the diabetic medication). Reassured, Clare gave Cassie the go-ahead. She explained the principles of the 800-calorie diet, discussed what foods Cassie could eat and those she couldn't. She offered regular email or phone support.

Cassie had no idea whether she would be able to stick to what sounded like a tough regime but she had two powerful motivating forces. Firstly, Grace. She didn't want her little girl growing up with a mum who was ill and incapacitated. Secondly, she had hit rock-bottom. "I had nothing to lose," she says.

What surprised her was that it didn't take long to get into a new habit. The first few days were tough – "it was like my stomach was eating itself" – but she swiftly got into a routine that worked for her. Lots of protein and vegetables, no refined carbohydrates. In the evening she would eat a smaller portion of what her husband was eating – a stir-fry or a salad.

Amazingly, after just a week the hunger ended. For the first time in her life she was no longer obsessed by food. It was a revelation.

Within two weeks she was able to stop her insulin and metformin. She didn't need them because her blood sugars had returned to normal. And they've stayed that way.

She stayed on the diet for eight weeks and lost just over 20kg (44lb). "I feel amazing. I don't think about food any more. I'm full of energy. Happy. I really do think I have been given another chance at life. I feel in control for the first time."

A couple of months after stopping medication she sent an email to say that after years of trying, she was pregnant again.

"I had a conversation with my midwife who said that some studies have shown that polycystic ovaries, which is what I have, can be caused by high amounts of insulin in the blood… She thinks that I got pregnant because I was able to come off my insulin. So I cannot thank you enough because not only have you freed me from food and put me back in charge of my own life, but you have also helped me to make a little miracle possible – which I never thought would happen."

Stress – the powerful role it has to play

As Cassie clearly demonstrates, food is tied up with how we feel. Emotions like stress, anger, fear and anxiety make us reach for the biscuit tin, which in turn will make our blood sugar go haywire.

Bereavement, divorce, work stress, redundancy – the more people I talked to for this book, the more I realised how much our emotions are linked to blood sugar. Almost everyone could date their problems back to emotional upheaval.

Over a century ago, Henry Maudsley, one of the founders of modern psychiatry, noted that blood sugar problems often followed sudden trauma. He reported the story of a soldier who, upon discovering that his wife was having an affair, immediately developed type 2 diabetes.[16] More recently, Walter Cannon, a scientist based at Harvard and the man who first came up with the term "fight or flight response", found that cats' blood sugar rose when they were frightened or stressed.[17]

So what is happening? Negative and stressful emotions such as anger or frustration or sadness drive up levels of stress hormones in the body like adrenaline and cortisol. These hormones are part of our "fight or flight" response, designed to help us survive in times of crisis by making glucose readily available to use as fuel. A study of non-diabetic bungee jumpers found that the stress of the jump caused blood sugar levels to rise significantly. This is just what you want if you're non-diabetic, but not if you have problems with blood sugar control.

Stress-related hormones make muscles and tissues more insulin-resistant. They stimulate the liver to release more sugar into the blood, prevent the pancreas from making insulin, and block insulin's ability to get sugar into cells.

This whole scenario feeds frustration, sadness and anger. To cheer yourself up – you eat more.

> *"The father we knew had disappeared in a fog of depression, embarrassment, lack of confidence and pain."*

Anthony and Ian Whitington didn't realise their father, Geoff, had fallen into a diabetes-related depression until it was almost too late. He had been diagnosed when he was 50. "He just took it on as yet another illness," recalls Anthony, "and so did we." They knew that he was on medication for high cholesterol and blood pressure. "But the diabetes news was a bit of a non-event. He didn't announce it. It just seemed like more pills to take."

Geoff's doctor could have urged him to change, but he didn't. He played it down. He told Geoff that this was something he could live with, something he could manage.

Busy doctors have developed a form of "learned helplessness". They know that standard dietary advice is rarely listened to or followed. So they watch the weight pile on and add more medication with a sense of resignation.

Geoff began a low-fat diet in a rather half-hearted way, but he didn't see much change and soon started eating in secret. Fast food may have been slowly killing him but it was also his way of cheering himself up. He'd go to McDonald's and hide the wrappers before he got home. At which point he would sit down to an evening meal as though he had not eaten since lunchtime. His wife Marion – who was trying to cook him healthier meals at home – had no idea that he was eating for two.

Eleven years after diagnosis he had an ulcer on his right foot, and a collapsed arch on the left one. Both can lead to amputation. He had neuropathy in his fingers – he could touch hot things and not notice. He was becoming reclusive. "The father we knew had disappeared in a fog of depression, embarrassment, lack of confidence and pain," says Anthony.

Anthony, who works in finance, and his brother Ian, a documentary maker, decided to stage an intervention. They came up with a plan to film their dad. They told him they were making a documentary about type 2 diabetes but what they were really doing was trying to get him interested in life again. "Initially he just played along with it, thinking it was just another one of our mad projects," laughs Anthony.

The result is an incredibly moving – and funny – film called "Fixing Dad". Geoff is now diabetes-free.

His readings used to be sky high. Now they are bouncing along in the normal range.

How did Geoff do it? His sons put him on a very low-calorie diet and asked him to take a photograph on his phone of every meal (making him accountable for everything he ate). They weaned him off his traditional meals and introduced him to new ingredients.

There were stand-up arguments in the supermarket – "There was a lot of high tension, a lot of arguments; we are all stubborn" – but he lost 18lb (8kg) in the first two weeks.

Geoff's sons had researched the evidence on rapid weight loss and how it can reverse diabetes and believed that they could turn their father's blood sugar problems – and his depression – around. "We really clung on to the idea that this was something potentially reversible. It was a real driving force. We told ourselves – it has fixed one person, maybe it can fix dad too. It was an important message – this can be *reversed*."

Gradually exercise became part of Geoff's new life. He took up cycling. The exercise made him feel good about himself. As part of the film his sons challenged him to new ideas – sky-diving, white-water rafting.

As well as losing weight – 84lb (38kg) – Geoff's mood gradually improved. "He is totally different now," says Anthony. "His aura, the way he projects himself; he has self-belief. He believes he can do things." So much so he has become a diabetes champion. The man who spent the last decade sitting at home now goes into companies and tells staff how to fix themselves.

Interestingly, Geoff had spent most of his career as a night-time security guard. A study in 2010 tested nine healthy adults to see what effect sleep deprivation has on insulin resistance.[18]

On one night, individuals were allowed to sleep for up to 8.5 hours (11pm – 7.30am). On another night, sleep was only permitted for four hours (1am – 5am). The actual average sleep times were seven hours 34 minutes and three hours 46 minutes respectively.

The results show that cutting sleep on one occasion was enough to increase insulin resistance. The internal production of sugar was higher, and clearance of glucose into muscle cells was lower in the sleep-deprived state.

Less than four hours sleep is not much sleep. But then again, increased insulin resistance was seen in individuals after just one night of sleep deprivation. It's possible that less extreme sleep deprivation over long periods of time also poses hazards for the body.

Later on in the book I will give you some techniques to manage stress.

Chapter four

GOING LOW-CARB

In chapter one, I explained why so many experts now believe that the obsession with "low-fat everything" helped fuel an over-consumption of cheap and easily digestible carbohydrates, which in turn helped feed the recent surge in obesity.

Easily digestible carbohydrates include all forms of sugars (the ones in fizzy drinks are among the worst offenders), many processed foods (sugars are now added to a huge range of foods), as well as crackers, cakes, breakfast cereals and even rice, pasta and bread.

Despite this, the standard advice for type 2 diabetics continues to be "Eat a low-fat diet". Diabetics are told to try and cut down on sugar, but to base their meals on starchy foods like potatoes, rice and pasta. Bread is encouraged, as are breakfast cereals. I was recently in a London teaching hospital, chatting to a 55-year-old man who was about to have his leg amputated because of type 2 diabetes. When I asked him what was offered for breakfast, he said, "I had a choice of white bread or cornflakes."

Twenty years ago you could have been forgiven for feeding diabetics this sort of food. But since then there have been literally dozens of studies that have shown again and again that this is not the way to go.

A recent review of 20 randomised controlled trials involving more than 3000 type 2 diabetics found that if you want to lose weight, improve your cholesterol and improve your blood sugar control, then your best bet is a low-carb, Mediterranean diet. It's a diet that is moderately high in fat and low in highly processed carbohydrates.[19]

What is a "Mediterranean diet"?

The Mediterranean diet has become incredibly popular since studies showed it can significantly cut your risk of heart disease, type 2 diabetes and possibly Alzheimer's. It is not a diet that most people associate with the Med. There is no pizza or pasta. Instead, it is a diet that emphasises the importance of eating fruit, vegetables, oily fish, nuts and olive oil. Yoghurt and cheese are warmly embraced. As is a glass of red wine at the end of the day (though this is optional). There are carbs in this diet, but the sort that your body takes longer to break down and absorb. That means legumes (beans, pulses, lentils), not pasta, rice or potatoes. I think it is a fantastically healthy and tasty way to eat. It takes many of the best features of a low-carb diet and makes them more palatable. I go into much more detail about how to Mediterraneanise your diet later in the book. Indeed, what I call the "M Plan" is the crux of the Blood Sugar Diet.

After 30 years as a family doctor David Unwin had become increasingly puzzled – and gloomy – about his patients.

"I couldn't understand why more and more of them were coming into the surgery overweight and with type 2 diabetes, sometimes decades earlier than they used to," he explains. "I didn't know how to help them. More often than not I started them on medication."

Then one day a former diabetes patient turned up – free of the disease. "She mystified me. But I am always fascinated by stories of success so I asked her what she had done."

She replied, "You're not going to like this doctor." She had read about the benefits of a low-carb, high-fat diet and given it a go.

Dr Unwin did some research and soon became convinced that part of the problem for type 2 diabetics is that their metabolism can no longer deal with sugar. "It's become almost like a poison," he says. The obvious answer is cut back, not just on sugar but foods that rapidly turn into sugars when they enter your body.

Putting patients on a low-carb diet is still viewed by many doctors as verging on the faddy, so it was against the advice of colleagues that he decided to do a small trial. He recruited 19 patients who had type 2 diabetes or prediabetes and gave them a very simple diet sheet.

"Reduce starchy carbohydrates a lot (remember they are just concentrated sugar)," it reads. "If possible, cut out the white stuff like bread, pasta, rice. As for sugar – cut it out altogether, although it will be in the blueberries, strawberries and raspberries you are allowed to eat freely."

Instead, patients were encouraged to eat more protein, butter, full-fat yoghurt and olive oil: "EATING LOTS OF VEG WITH PROTEIN AND FATS LEAVES YOU PROPERLY FULL IN A WAY THAT LASTS," he wrote in capital letters.

In a spirit of solidarity, and because he wanted to lose some weight himself, Dr Unwin went on the diet. His wife, a clinical psychologist, worked with patients on the emotional aspects of weight loss. Crucially, rather than focusing on the downsides to type 2 diabetes, she helped patients to focus on the positive aspects of losing weight.

One of the patients dropped out early on, but the others found it simple and easy to stick to. They started out with an average weight of 100kg (220lb) and over the eight months of the trial lost over 9kg (20lb), much of it around the waist.[20]

Seven patients came off medication and most reported improved energy and wellbeing, which in turn meant they were more inclined to do exercise.

By the end only two of the 19 still had raised

blood sugars and even those two had seen a huge improvement.

There were also big improvements in blood pressure and cholesterol levels, despite the fact that his patients were now eating far more eggs and butter.

Dr Unwin was struck by just how keen his patients were to take control of their own lives and not rely on him to solve their problems. People who were not officially part of the trial asked to join in.

"I was worried what other doctors in the practice would think," he recalls. "I thought they might think I was buying into something that was seen as mumbo-jumbo. But the success of the patients emboldened me."

The patients who lost the weight have kept it off and more have gone through his programme, saving his practice over £15,000 a year on its diabetes drug budget. The number of obese patients in his practice has also fallen substantially. "It is all about seeing the potential in people. Giving them a choice," says Dr Unwin.

Do you crave carbs? Are you addicted?

Try this short quiz about your relationship with carbohydrates.

Do you get an instant reward or "hit" as soon as you eat sweet, starchy or refined foods?	YES / NO
Do you eat five or more portions of carbohydrates most days (in addition to sweet things, this includes pasta, bread, potatoes, rice and cereals)?	YES / NO
Do you often drink sweetened or flavoured drinks (including fruit juice and artificially sweetened drinks)?	YES / NO
Do you often snack or graze between meals?	YES / NO
Do you eat three or more portions of fruit a day?	YES / NO
Do you usually have generous portions of carbohydrate-rich foods with most of your meals, getting over 30% of your calories from starchy and refined carbohydrates, including bread, pasta, potatoes, rice and cereals? (Brown versions of all these still count as starch!)	YES / NO
Do you often eat to make yourself feel better, for example when you are disappointed, under pressure or have had an argument?	YES / NO
Are you eating large portions?	YES / NO
Do you often feel unsatisfied, even soon after finishing a meal?	YES / NO
Does the sight, smell or thought of food often stimulate you to eat, even if you have just finished a meal or are not hungry?	YES / NO
Do you often lose control and eat much more than you meant to, particularly when eating snacks, junk food, or sweets? (May involve eating until uncomfortable, feeling sick or actually being sick.)	YES / NO
Do you often justify eating by thinking "Just this time", or "Later I will eat better/start the diet/burn it off"?	YES / NO

Is food much on your mind? Do you often find yourself thinking about food during the day?	YES / NO
Do you sometimes eat in secret?	YES / NO
Do you sometimes snack late at night or during the night?	YES / NO
Do you often feel guilty or ashamed about what you are eating, yet find yourself eating it again soon after?	YES / NO
Do you often crave carbohydrates or feel shaky, irritable, anxious or sweaty without them?	YES / NO

Add up the number of "Yes" answers and see which group you are in below:

0–3 You don't appear to be addicted.
    You can take it or leave it when it comes to eating carbs and probably have a fairly healthy attitude towards food.

4–8 You may be addicted to carbs.
    You like your carbs, but are probably managing to keep it in check. This may require a certain amount of self-control. At times you probably find this a bit of a challenge. The problem with carbs is that for many people, the more you eat, the more you want. It is a slippery slope.

9–13 Moderately addicted to carbs.
    You are eating considerably more than you know is good for you and are probably feeling bad about it. You are likely to be feeling hungry much of the time, preoccupied by food and at times struggling to control your cravings as a result of a degree of insulin resistance. You are probably at risk of developing diabetes, if you don't have it already. Worth getting regular health checks.

14–17 Severe addiction to carbs.
    Avoiding carbs is a real challenge for you. You are likely

to be constantly hungry, preoccupied by food, feeling bad and guilty about your eating. You are highly likely to have insulin resistance (metabolic syndrome). Given the amount of carbs you are eating and your unhealthy relationship to them, you're at significant risk of developing diabetes, if you don't have it already. Definitely worth getting regular health checks.

The truth about carbohydrates

I'm not saying all carbs are bad. Along with fats and proteins, carbs play an important role in our diet. The problem occurs when you eat too much of the wrong sort. Carbs broadly come in two main categories:

Easily digestible carbs
These are the sort that are rapidly absorbed by your body and which create an instant spike in blood sugar. These include not just the sugar you add to your tea or quaff in fizzy drinks, but also "natural sugars" such as honey, maple syrup, agave nectar, etc. Processed foods are stuffed full of sugars.

"Easily digestible carbs" also include starches like bread, rice, pasta and potatoes. This doesn't mean that rice and potatoes are evil, but don't pile your plate with them. Think of them more as a side dish than a staple and try to find alternatives.

Complex, unrefined carbs

These are the "good" type that contain lots of fibre, making them harder to absorb. Slow absorption is a good thing. Examples include vegetables, legumes and whole grains.

Unfortunately, genuine "whole grains" are hard to find. Most of the brown breads and cereals you buy, despite what it says on the packet, are not really "whole grains" but heavily processed. In some cases the manufacturers add extra sugar to brown bread to counteract the bitterness.

Easily digestible carbs are the "baddies" because they can cause blood sugar spikes and result in the over-production of insulin. But how can you tell whether you are eating good or bad carbs?

One way is by looking up its Glycaemic Index (GI) score. Foods are ranked from 0 to 100 (with sugar being 100). Unrefined carbohydrates normally have a low GI, meaning they cause blood sugar levels to rise slowly, helping you to feel fuller for longer. Refined carbohydrates, on the other hand, tend to have a high GI, which means they cause a rapid spike in blood sugar levels, which then crash. This will encourage you to eat more.

GI is a measure of the speed at which your blood sugars rise. But the size of the spike in blood sugars is not just the result of the type of food you eat but also the amount you eat. Your portion size.

The way to measure the overall impact of a particular

food on your blood sugar is by calculating its Glycaemic Load (GL):

$$GL = (GI \times \text{the amount of carbohydrate}) \text{ divided by } 100$$

An apple, for example, has a GI score of 40. It contains about 15g of carbs so its GL =

$$(40 \times 15)/100 = 6$$

If you think this sounds complicated, you're right. It is. To get your head round it properly I recommend going to the University of Sydney's website, as they have been at the forefront of GI research for over 20 years: http://www.glycemicindex.com/

The Sydney researchers say, as a rule of thumb, you should be wary of carbs with a GI over 55 or a GL over 20.

Foods with a high GI/GL score include white bread, cornflakes, white rice, potatoes and bagels.

Those with low GI/GL include most vegetables, nuts, seeds, whole grains (millet, oat, rye), mushrooms and most fruits.

Below are a few examples taken from the glycemicindex website:

Food	Glycaemic Index (under 55 is OK)	Glycaemic Load (over 20 is high)
Cooked carrots	33	2
Lentils	22	4
An apple	40	6
Apple juice	44	13
Mashed potato	83	17
White pasta (cooked)	61	29
Wholemeal pasta (cooked)	58	29
White rice	72	30
Brown rice	48	20
Bagel	69	24

As you can see, some of the foods we've been urged to fill up on, such as pasta and rice, have a very high GL. Switching to lower GL versions of these staples can produce significant improvements in blood sugar control.

GI and GL are useful, but only up to a point. Trying to base what you eat entirely on GI charts will prove stressful and complicated because, among others things, they don't take into account two other hugely important food groups, fats and proteins. I prefer a much simpler approach, which I detail later.

A word on fructose

One form of sugar that has been demonised above all others in recent years is fructose. So what is it and why does it have such a bad reputation?

Fructose is a form of sugar that is commonly found in fruit and ordinary table sugar. It is, notoriously, also found in high-quantities in corn syrup, which has in the last few decades been added to many processed foods and carbonated drinks.

Fructose is incredibly sweet, but the main problem with it is the way it is treated by your body. Unlike glucose, which can be taken up by any cell, fructose has to be processed by the liver. In small amounts that is fine, but in the quantities we consume today it leads to liver overload.

One of the things that the liver does with excess fructose is turn it into fat. Load it with enough fructose and you get a "fatty liver".

To cut down on fructose you will need to read the food labels carefully – it can be called "high fructose corn syrup", "glucose-fructose syrup" or even "isoglucose".

Fruit also contains fructose. So while it is good to eat a certain amount of fresh fruit, whole, and with the skin on, you should try to minimise your consumption of juices and smoothies, which have had the fibre stripped out. A small glass of orange juice has twice the sugar, twice the calories and half the fibre of an orange.

So fibre is still seen as a good thing? It sounds so 1970s...

Yes, eating more fibre is one other way to slow the rate at which your body absorbs sugar. Lack of fibre in our diet is a leading cause of the current diabesity epidemic. The average adult eats about 15g of fibre a day and you should be eating at least twice that. Studies suggest that contemporary hunter-gatherer peoples (whose diet is closest to that of our ancient ancestors) eat at least 100g per day, maybe more.

Fibre not only slows the absorption of sugars, but, because it passes largely undigested through the small bowel, it also provides food for the trillions of healthy bacteria that lurk in the large bowel. There are thousands of different species of bacteria living in your gut, as rich an ecosystem as you will find in a rainforest, and having the right mix is important for your health. Eating plenty of fibre helps the "good guys" thrive.

You can get reasonable amounts of extra fibre by eating more beans, chickpeas, bulgur wheat, artichokes, leafy green vegetables, broccoli, cauliflower, carrots, cabbage, oats, nuts, raspberries, blackberries, apples and pears.

Chapter five

THE RETURN OF THE VLCD (THE VERY LOW-CALORIE DIET)

I have explained why cutting out easily digestible carbs will help reduce hunger and blood sugar surges. Now I want to address some of the anxieties you might have about rapid weight loss before going on to look at the Blood Sugar Diet itself.

Most of us have heard, countless times, that if you lose weight fast you will put it all back on even faster. It is a key part of dieting folklore.

I heard a leading nutritionist on the radio the other day saying with complete confidence, "Very low-calorie diets are really bad for you and they don't work. There's absolutely no benefit to doing them or fasting or detoxing. It's just wishful thinking."

A few years ago I would have agreed, and if you had asked me what I thought of rapid weight loss I would have said it was a terrible idea. Everyone knows, I'd have said, about the dangers of yo-yo dieting. Everyone knows that the only successful way to lose weight in the long run is to do it gradually, sensibly, cutting your calories slowly, aiming to lose around 1–2lb (500g–1kg) a week. But that was before I took a serious look at the science. And it turns out that much of what I used to accept as "proven" is actually based on myth.

There is certainly a rich history of faddy crash diets out there, from the lemonade fast to the cabbage soup diet. The latest versions include juicing and cleansing diets, promising you can lose "7lb in 7 Days". Now some of these diets do deliver impressive weight loss. At least initially. The problem is that most of them are so boring that they become impossibly difficult to sustain. What's more, some don't have enough protein in them, so lead to muscle loss (you need to maintain your muscle mass to keep your metabolic rate up and to help mop up sugar surges).

The other problem is that the scales lie.

Just as jockeys are able to shed pounds two days before a race by fasting, at the start of a VLCD what you are losing is mainly water, not fat. The initial results are fabulous but when you stop, the water piles back on, and so does the weight.

One of the most notorious of the crash diets was the Last Chance Diet, promoted in the 1970s by osteopath Robert Linn. Linn, who at one point weighed 235lb (107kg), became interested in diets after developing heart palpitations in his mid-forties. He began experimenting with high-protein liquid diets, lost a lot of weight and then started up a weight loss clinic. He subsequently published his book, which sold well over 2.5 million copies.

Along with his bestselling book you could also buy his miraculous "liquid protein diet", Prolinn. Prolinn provided less than 400 calories a day, but it really seemed to work. There were numerous personal endorsements by celebrities who assured the public that they could lose up to 10lb (4.5kg) a week.

After initial success, however, things fell apart. The Last Chance Diet began to live up to its name. There were reports of deaths and the FDA was asked to investigate. Although some of the fatalities seem to have been people who already had advanced heart disease and might have died anyway, there was evidence in a few cases that the diet itself might be causing damage to the heart through what was identified as "protein-calorie malnutrition".

The thing about protein is that it is not a source of fuel like fat or carbohydrates, but primarily a source of amino acids. Among other things, these help build muscle, and are only used as a source of fuel when your fat and carbohydrate stores start to run down.

Unlike fat or carbohydrates, protein is not stored by the body. If you don't get enough in your diet your body will break down your muscles to top up your amino acids. The longer you go without, the more damage you do. That is why it is so important that whatever diet you go on you make sure that it is rich in high-quality protein.

The problem for Last Chance dieters who used Prolinn, or other copycat products, was that the protein in those sachets came largely from collagen, a low-quality protein that they got from the tendons, ligaments and skin of animals. Living on nothing but chemically pre-digested cowhide and tendons, scavenged from slaughterhouse animals and then enhanced with artificial flavourings and sweeteners, was never likely to end well.

Not surprisingly, the Last Chance Diet and others of its type have cast a long shadow over the reputation of VLCDs.

But as some of America's leading obesity experts pointed out in a review article in the *New England Journal of Medicine*[21] in 2013, it is a myth that slow and gradual weight loss is more effective than rapid weight loss, despite the fact that it has been repeated in text books for decades.

The authors point out (and the article is really worth reading) that numerous trials have shown that "more rapid and greater initial weight loss is associated with lower body weight at the end of long-term follow-up". In other words, if you want to diet successfully it can be better to lose weight quickly than slowly.

A recent Australian study[22] backs up these claims. In this trial they took 200 obese volunteers and put half of them on a VLCD (less than 800 calories a day). Their goal was to lose 12.5% of their body weight within 12 weeks.

The other half were put on a low-fat diet, cutting their normal weekly intake by about 500 calories a day. They were given 36 weeks to achieve similar levels of weight loss as the rapid dieters.

There was a very high drop-out rate among the steady low-fat dieters: less than half made it to the end of the 36 weeks. It's not surprising: going low-fat is hard and people often get frustrated by the slow rate of progress. By comparison, more than 80% of people assigned to the rapid weight loss programme achieved their goal. On the downside, one person in the rapid weight loss group developed acute cholecystitis (inflammation of the gall bladder) which may have been due to the diet.

Katrina Purcell, a dietician who led the study, said, "Across the world, guidelines recommend gradual weight loss for the treatment of obesity, reflecting the widely held belief that fast weight loss is more quickly regained. However, our results show that achieving a weight loss target of 12.5% is more likely, and drop-out is lower, if losing weight is done quickly."

She thinks that losing weight fast motivates dieters to stick with their programme because they see rapid results. A VLCD also means less carbohydrates, which forces the body to burn fat more quickly.

Both groups were then followed for another three years. Although most put some weight back on, the amounts were similar in the two groups.

Commenting on this study, Dr Corby Martin and Professor Kishore Gadde from Pennington Biomedical Research Center, Baton Rouge, wrote, "This study... indicates that for weight loss, a slow and steady approach does not win the race, and the myth that rapid weight loss is associated with rapid weight regain is no more true than Aesop's fable."

Professor Nick Finer, a consultant endocrinologist and bariatric physician at University College London Hospitals, also commented: "This study shows clearly that rapid weight loss does not lead to faster weight regain, but importantly can be a better approach since more people achieved their target loss, and fewer dropped out of treatment. If we couple these findings with those from other groups that have shown dramatic and immediate improvements in diabetes and blood pressure with rapid weight loss (i.e. the Newcastle group), this should be part of NHS approaches to treatment."

Professor Taylor says there is a world of difference between a crash diet and what he's recommending. "A crash diet has an unplanned element to it: where you desperately cut out all food and only drink green juice before going back to what you did before. That is an unplanned crash. We have a planned approach to eating. Reduce food intake. Keep it low for eight weeks. Then have a stepped return to eating less than you used to. Often people want to keep dieting for longer. It is because they feel so well. Almost to a person they say 'I feel 10 years younger.' What they are wary of is going back on to the stuff that used to poison them – too much food."

His colleague, Professor Mike Lean of Glasgow University, is also adamant that for many people rapid weight loss is the way to go. "Doing it slowly is a torture.

Contrary to the belief of dieticians – people who lose weight more quickly, more emphatically, are more likely to keep it off in the long term. Dieticians are still teaching that you should lose weight slowly to keep it off. Wrong. Wrong. Wrong. This is based largely on the very old 1960s low-calorie diet – people who went on crash diets with no maintenance programme. If you have no maintenance programme of course you put the weight back on."

There are people who should be cautious about following such a low-calorie diet, and I list them in the "Before you start" section on page 124. But for many it could prove a pathway back to health.

The people who've tried the Blood Sugar Diet have certainly been impressed. Heidi, for example, wrote in to say, "I lost 25 pounds in a year on Weight Watchers and 28 pounds in eight weeks on the Blood Sugar Diet; I was less satisfied on Weight Watchers too."

Eight hundred calories for 8 weeks has not only helped reverse most cases of type 2 diabetes, it has also proved to be extremely effective at helping people with pre-diabetes from progressing on to diabetes.

A recent study, the largest of its kind, backs up this claim. The Preview study[23] was set up some time ago to find the best ways to stem the apparently inexorable rise of type 2 diabetes.

For this study 2,326 overweight men and women from eight countries (Britain, Denmark, Finland, Holland, Bulgaria, Spain, New Zealand and Australia) with pre-diabetes were asked to go on an 800-calorie diet for eight weeks, with the aim of losing 8 per cent of their body weight.

To the researchers' great surprise, they did far better than that, losing an average of 24lb in 8 weeks. Professor Jennie Brand-Miller of the University of Sydney, one of the lead researchers, told me that she was particularly pleased by the effect this had on their blood sugar levels. "In many cases", she said, "their blood glucose is back to healthy levels and their pre-diabetes has disappeared."

She also told me that although the volunteers found living on 800 calories tough to start with, most of them soon adapted and stopped feeling hungry. And when they lost weight, they became more active, which added to the benefits.

Other common myths about rapid weight loss

"There's no point in doing a rapid weight loss diet because within a few days of starting you will go into starvation mode, your metabolic rate will slow and your weight loss will stop."

False. Fear of going into "starvation mode" is common and seems to be based, in part, on the Minnesota starvation experiment, carried out during World War Two. In this study,[24] 36 male volunteers spent six months on a low-calorie diet consisting largely of potatoes, turnips, bread and macaroni. The study was done to help scientists understand how to treat victims of mass starvation in Europe.

Not fat to begin with, the volunteers became incredibly skinny and their metabolic rates slowed down. Obviously, though, this was an extreme situation.

A more recent experiment on the effects of short-term calorie restriction produced very different results. In this study,[25] 11 healthy volunteers were asked to live on nothing but water for 84 hours (just under four days). The researchers found that the volunteers' metabolic rate actually went *up* while they were fasting. By Day 3 it had risen, on average, by 14%. One reason for this may have been the rise in certain hormones, known to burn fat.

In the long run your metabolic rate will slow down, however quickly or slowly you lose weight, simply because you are now no longer carrying the equivalent of a large, heavy suitcase full of fat wherever you go. That is why it is important to keep your metabolic rate up by doing strength exercises (see later) and keeping active as your weight drops.

"It is better to set 'realistic' weight loss goals because if you are too ambitious you are doomed to fail."

False. We're always told to be realistic, and many people would say that trying to lose a lot of weight really fast is unrealistic. Yet research suggests that people who set out with more ambitious goals tend to lose more weight. In a study[26] nearly 2000 overweight men and women were asked about their goals before they started on a weight loss programme. They were followed for two years, by which time those with "less realistic goals" had lost the most weight.

"If I cut my calories dramatically I will feel hungry all the time and end up crashing out of the diet."

False. Many of the people I've talked to who have followed a VLCD say that hunger typically disappears within 48 hours. Some people get problems, like headaches, but these are often due to dehydration. You are missing out on the fluid you would normally take in with your food, plus, as you burn fat you lose water. If you don't drink enough, your blood pressure can drop and you may feel faint. To anticipate and avoid this you should increase your fluid intake – I will write more on this in the next chapter.

SECTION II

THE BLOOD SUGAR DIET (BSD)

Chapter six

THE THREE CORE PRINCIPLES OF THE BSD & WHAT TO DO BEFORE YOU START

So far I've explained the background to the current obesity crisis, underlined the dangers that come with prediabetes and diabetes, introduced you to the science behind the VLCD approach and, hopefully, inspired you with stories of people who have already succeeded with it.

Time to get on to the practicalities of the diet itself. It is a bold and radical diet, one that involves eating 800 calories a day for up to eight weeks. It will help you get rid of your tummy (visceral) fat fast. Once your visceral fat levels start to drop (and this happens within days), the fat clogging up your liver will also begin to melt away like snow under a hot sun. Within weeks both prediabetics and type 2 diabetics should see their blood sugar levels falling back towards normal. This will set you on course for a leaner, healthier future.

But this is not just a one-off weight loss programme to be done and dusted in a matter of weeks. It is part of a lifestyle programme built on three core principles intended to support you not only while you are on the diet, but also, crucially, when you have finished and are moving on to the next stage in your life. Understanding and applying them is important for long-term success.

So here they are, the three core principles of the BSD.

1. Going Mediterranean

I am going to introduce you to a Mediterranean-style, low-carb eating plan (M Plan, for short). This is a tasty and healthy way of living. It is low in starchy, easily digestible carbs, but packed full of disease-fighting vitamins and flavonoids. It is rich in olive oil, fish, nuts, fruit and vegetables, but also contains lots of lovely things that down the years we have been told not to eat, such as full-fat yoghurt and eggs.

In huge, randomised studies researchers have found that not only do people get multiple health benefits from a Mediterranean style of eating but they are good at sticking to it (unlike those who go on a low-fat diet) because they find it easy and enjoyable.[27]

Although it is derived from the eating habits of people living in Mediterranean countries, you can apply the principles of Med-style eating to a wide range of different cuisines, from Chinese or Indian through to Mexican or Scandanavian.

The menus in this book all follow the principles of the M Plan. In the next section I will outline the changes you need to make to your diet to improve what I call your "M score", and your long-term health. Before that I will give a brief description of the other two key "pillars" of the Blood Sugar Diet, "Getting Active" and "Sorting Your Head", both of which will be fleshed out more fully in chapters eight and nine.

2. Getting active

We all know how important being more active is, yet few of us find the time or inclination to go on regular runs or visits to the gym. If you are thinking to yourself, "You must be joking, I can't possibly become more active while cutting my calories", then be reassured. The activity programme I outline in chapter eight is not going to leave you tired or hungry. It should improve your mood and make the diet easier.

Being more active is also the best way to reverse insulin resistance, which lies at the heart of most blood sugar problems.

In "Before You Start" (see page 124) I will give you a simple way to assess your current level of fitness and show you how this will improve over the eight weeks of the diet.

You will start by standing up more and increasing the amount that you walk.

You will also need to do a set of resistance, strength-building exercises, which you will start on Day 1 of the diet and build over the eight weeks. No special equipment required.

Finally, you will be introduced to one of the biggest breakthroughs in sports science in the last decade. It is a cardio programme that in a few weeks can significantly improve your aerobic fitness, the strength of your heart and lungs. The programme outlined in this book has been specifically designed for diabetics and those who are currently not very fit, and you will be pleased to hear that it does not involve hours of jogging. In fact it only requires *a few minutes a week*. It is optional, but it is very effective and it is something I now do on a regular basis.

3. Sorting out your head

The final principle is about getting your head in the right place – learning how to de-stress and reduce impulsive eating.

We all know how easy it is, when things go wrong, to reach for the biscuit tin or the reassuring slab of high-calorie cake. Well, this is the stress hormone, cortisol, in action. As well as driving "comfort eating", cortisol makes your body more insulin-resistant, which makes you hungry. All good reasons to get your stress levels down.

While making a science documentary about the brain not long ago (*The Truth about Personality*), I investigated different ways to reduce stress and build resilience and the one I found most effective was mindfulness. It's a modern take on meditation, something that has been practised by all the great religions.

In recent years mindfulness has become incredibly fashionable among celebrities, business leaders and athletes. The reason is: it works. A few short sessions of mindfulness done each week should be enough to reduce stress and anxiety.[28] I was sceptical before I began doing it three years ago, but I have now made it part of my life.

So these are the three core principles that will support you through the BSD and which I hope you'll maintain when you finish it. Before moving on to the details of the BSD itself, let's look in a bit more detail at the Mediterranean diet, and how you can Mediterraneanise your eating habits.

The "M Plan"

There have been numerous studies providing overwhelming evidence of the benefits of Mediterranean-style eating, one of the most impressive being the PREDIMED trial (Prevención con Dieta Mediterránea), which began in 2003 and is still ongoing. For this trial Spanish researchers recruited over 7400 people, many of them type 2 diabetics, and randomly allocated them to a Mediterranean or a low-fat diet.[29]

Both groups were encouraged to eat lots of fresh fruit, vegetables and legumes (such as beans, lentils and peas). They were also discouraged from sugary drinks, cakes, sweets or pastries and from eating too much processed meat (like bacon or salami).

The main difference between the two diets was that those allocated to the Mediterranean diet were asked to eat plenty of eggs, nuts and oily fish and use lots of olive oil. They were also encouraged to eat some chocolate, preferably dark and made with more than 50% cocoa, and were allowed to enjoy the occasional glass of wine with their evening meal.

The low-fat group, by contrast, were encouraged to eat low-fat dairy products and eat lots of starchy foods, like bread, potatoes, pasta and rice.

The result? Well, it turned out that those on the Mediterranean diet were 30% less likely to die from a heart attack or stroke. Subsequent studies have shown even more health benefits (more on these shortly).

Dr Mario Kratz, a nutritional scientist at the Fred Hutchinson Cancer Research Center in Seattle who has looked at lots of studies on low- versus high-fat dairy, says, "None of the research suggests low-fat dairy is better." In fact, plenty of studies have found that eating full-fat dairy is *less* likely to lead to obesity.[30]

In the Predimed study this certainly seemed to be the case. Despite significantly cutting their fat intake the low-fat group started to add more fat around their waists. After 5 years their waist size had increased by an average of ½ inch.[31]

On the other hand those adding healthy fats to their diet (which we recommend) reported feeling less hungry. As someone recently wrote to me, "As soon as I added walnuts, more olives or olive oil to my diet, the hunger stopped and my mind became clearer."

Commenting on the Predimed study, Professor Dariush Mozaffarian from the Friedman School of Nutrition Science & Policy at Tufts University, Boston, said: "We must abandon the myth that lower-fat, lower-calorie products lead to less weight gain… we ban whole milk but allow sugar-sweetened fat-free milk; we compel food manufacturers, retailers, and restaurants to remove healthy fats from meals and products while heavily marketing fat-reduced products of dubious health value; and mislead consumers to select foods based on total fat and calorie contents rather than actual health effects."

He went on to add, "We ignore this evidence – including these results from the PREDIMED trial – at our peril."

What is your M score?

(Adapted from "Primary prevention of cardiovascular disease with a mediterranean diet", Ramon Estruch et al).

Add a point for each "yes" answer. 10 or more is good.

1. Do you use olive oil as your main cooking fat and dressing?
2. Do you eat 2 or more portions of vegetables a day? (1 serving = 200g/7oz)
3. Do you eat 2 or more portions of fruit a day? (No points for sweet tropical fruits)
4. Do you eat less than 1 serving of processed meat a day? (1 serving = 100g/3.5oz)
5. Do you eat full-fat yoghurt at least 3 times a week?
6. Do you eat 3 or more servings of legumes – e.g. peas, beans, lentils – a week? (1 serving = 150g/5.25oz)
7. Do you eat 3 or more servings of whole grains a week? (1 serving = 150g/5.25oz)
8. Do you eat oily fish, prawns or shellfish 3 or more times a week? (100–150g/3.5–5.25oz fish)
9. Do you eat sweet treats like cakes, biscuits, etc less than 3 times a week?
10. Do you eat a serving of nuts (30g/1oz) 3 or more times a week?
11. Do you cook with garlic, onions and tomatoes at least 3 times a week?

12. Do you average around 7 glasses of wine or spirits a week?

13. Do you sit at the table to eat at least twice a day?

14. Do you drink sweet, fizzy beverages less than once a week?

Notes:

• Potatoes do not count as a vegetable

• Sweet tropical fruits include melon, grapes, pineapple and bananas

• Processed meat includes ham, bacon, sausages and salami

• Legumes include lentils and kidney beans

• Whole grains include quinoa, whole rye, bulgur wheat

• Nuts should be unsalted and include walnuts, almonds, cashew nuts and peanuts

• Drinking much more than 7 units of alcohol a week can be harmful

The impressive thing about the Mediterranean diet is just how widespread its benefits are. Not only does it cut your risk of heart disease and diabetes,[32] but according to a very recent finding women with a high M score have 68% less chance of developing breast cancer[33] than those on a low-fat diet. Consuming extra-virgin olive oil (the fresh squeezed juice of olives) seems to be particularly beneficial when it comes to cancer, perhaps because it contains compounds such as polyphenols which are known to be anti-inflammatory.

Tip: keep your oils in a cupboard as they degrade in sunlight.

The Mediterranean diet even seems to keep your brain in better shape. Evidence for this from the Predimed study, but also from a review article published in July 2016,[34] in which Dr Roy Hardman and colleagues from the Centre for Human Psychopharmacology in Melbourne, Australia looked at over a dozen studies published in the last fifteen years which measured the impact of the Mediterranean diet on people's brains.[35]

What they found was that the closer people stuck to a Mediterranean diet (the higher their M score) the less likely they were to show signs of cognitive decline (that's when you struggle to learn new things, remember or make decisions) and the less likely they were to develop Alzheimer's disease. The areas of the brain that seemed to get the most benefit from a Mediterranean diet were executive function (the part of your brain involved in decision making) and memory.

And it wasn't just the middle-aged or older people who got the benefit. Two of the studies which they looked at involved younger adults, and again those who had a higher M score did much better on computerised tests.

Finally, a brief note on alcohol. The Mediterranean diet includes a glass or two of wine with the evening meal. There have been endless arguments as to whether drinking moderate amounts of alcohol is healthy or not. The best way to find out would be to give alcohol to a group of non-drinkers and see what happens. Well, a research team in Israel has recently done just that.[36]

They took 224 teetotal diabetics and randomly allocated them to drinking either a medium-sized glass (150ml) of red wine, white wine or mineral water for their evening meal, every evening, for two years. The wine and water were provided free of charge and the empty bottles collected afterwards to make sure they really were drinking regularly.

So what happened? Well, red-wine drinkers will be delighted to hear it was the group drinking red wine who came out on top. They saw significant improvements in their cholesterol levels and the quality of their sleep. Some also had better blood sugar control.

Based on all of the above I've come up with a very simple guide on how to Mediterraneanise your diet, which diabetic and prediabetic patients have tried with considerable success.

The M Plan: what to eat to control your weight and your blood sugar

Firstly, cut right down on sugar, sugary treats, drinks and desserts. No more than once or twice a week and preferably less. We offer lots of recipes for healthy alternative foods below. You can use sugar substitutes like stevia and xylitol, but try to wean yourself off your sweet tooth.

Minimise or avoid the starchy "white stuff": bread, pasta, potatoes, rice. Be wary of "brown" alternatives: the extra fibre can be negligible. Brown rice is OK, but some wholemeal breads have added sugar.

Switch instead to quinoa, bulgur (cracked wheat), whole rye, whole-grain barley, wild rice and buckwheat. Legumes, such as lentils and kidney beans, are healthy and filling.

Avoid most breakfast cereals: they are usually full of sugar, even the ones that contain bran. Oats are good as long as they are not the instant sort.

Full-fat yoghurt is also good. Add berries, like blackberries, strawberries or blueberries, for flavour. Or a sprinkling of nuts.

Start the day with eggs: boiled, poached, scrambled or as an omelette – they'll keep you fuller for longer than cereal or toast. Delicious with smoked salmon, mushrooms and a sprinkle of chilli.

Snack on nuts: they are a great source of protein and fibre. Try to avoid salted or sweetened nuts, which can be moreish.

Eat more healthy fats and oils. Along with oily fish (salmon, tuna, mackerel), consume more olive oil. A splash makes vegetables taste better and improves the absorption of vitamins. Use olive, rapeseed or coconut oil for cooking.

Avoid margarine and use butter instead. Cheese in moderation is fine.

High-quality proteins to wolf down include: oily fish, prawns, chicken, turkey, pork, beef and, of course, eggs. Other protein-rich foods: soya, edamame beans, Quorn, hummus. Processed meats (bacon, salami, sausages) should be eaten only a few times a week.

Eat plenty of different coloured veg (from dark leafy greens to bright-red and yellow peppers. Add sauces and flavouring – lemon, butter or olive oil, salt, pepper, garlic, chilli, gravy.

Avoid too many sweet fruits: berries, apples or pears are fine, but sweet tropical fruits such as mango, pineapple, melon and bananas are full of sugar.

Have a drink, but not too many. Try to average no more than one to two units a day (a small glass of wine or shot of spirits is 1.5 units) and cut back on beer – it's rich in carbs, which is why it's known as "liquid toast".

What's rather depressing is that although most doctors are aware of the research I've just quoted, many don't feel comfortable putting it into practice. A recent survey of 236 cardiologists and internal medicine physicians at a large US academic medical centre found that while all of them think nutrition is important, only 13% felt sufficiently well informed to talk to patients about it. Most admitted to spending less than three minutes advising their patients about diet or exercise.[37]

Again, though most of them knew that a Mediterranean diet can cut the risk of heart disease and stroke, few were aware that in randomised trials low-fat diets have failed to do so, which may be why so many still recommend a low-fat diet.

As the Harvard School of Public Health points out on its website[38] the final nail in the low-fat coffin should have been the Women's Health Initiative (WHI) Dietary Modification Trial. In this trial, which began in 1993, 48,000 women were randomly allocated to either a low-fat diet or to continuing as normal. After eight years the trial was stopped. There were no differences in rates of cancer, heart disease or weight between the two groups.

This is not a licence to guzzle pints of cream and have lots of fried food, but it does mean that healthy fats like olive oil and nuts can be eaten without guilt.

Before you start

Confucius, the Chinese philosopher, pointed out more than 2000 years ago, "Success depends upon previous preparation, and without such preparation there is sure to be failure." Or as the actor Will Smith put it more recently, "I've always considered myself to be just average talent and what I have is a ridiculous, insane obsessiveness for practice and preparation."

The first thing I recommend you do is read this book all the way through to the end. The temptation is to dive in but it is important to get a full overview before you start. It is also important to be able to explain to your doctor what it is you are trying to achieve and the science behind it.

Talk to your doctor

I've been a bit critical of doctors in the early section of this book, but I am not anti-doctors, by any means. Most are very open-minded. Some of my best friends are doctors. I'm married to one. My son is training to become one. So do talk to yours before starting.

If you are on medication it is particularly important to have their buy-in as they should be involved in monitoring and tapering off your medicines. While many doctors will be delighted that you are taking responsibility for your health, some may be unimpressed. Work on them. Have a bet with them that you will succeed. It will give you motivation, and your success may inspire them to recommend it to other patients.

Caution – discuss with your doctor if any of the following apply:

- You have a history of eating disorders

- You are on insulin or a diabetic medication other than metformin – you may need to plan how you reduce your medication to avoid too fast a drop in blood sugar

- You are on blood pressure tablets – you may have to reduce or come off them

- You have moderate or severe retinopathy – you should have an extra screening within six months of reducing or reversing the diabetes

- You are pregnant or breastfeeding

- You have a significant psychiatric disorder

- You are taking warfarin

- You have epilepsy

- You have a significant medical condition

Don't go on the diet if:

- You are under 18

- Your BMI is below 21

- You are recovering from surgery or you are generally frail

You can get useful information, including a fact sheet that Professor Taylor has written for healthcare professionals and which you can download and give to your doctor from the Newscastle University website: http://www.ncl.ac.uk/magres/research/diabetes/reversal.htm

As he points out, you should confirm with your doctor that you really are a type 2 diabetic. There are other, rarer forms, like pancreatic, monogenic or slow onset type 1 diabetes that will not respond in the same way to weight loss.

Getting to know yourself – tests you should do

I love finding out more about my own body and I find it fascinating monitoring the changes that occur when I go through a new exercise regime or try new food. You can keep records of your results in a diary, or log into thebloodsugardiet.com where you can store your data safely and anonymously. The site will also provide useful updates on the latest science and a wealth of other information.

Another reason to keep a diary, electronic or otherwise, is to monitor exactly what you eat and drink. Some of those who have successfully followed this diet used the MyFitnessPal website to monitor calories and other nutrient inputs. But a diary is only of value if it is honest and accurate. A few years ago I made a film in which we asked an overweight actress to keep a food diary for a couple of weeks. At the same time we gave her a drink containing something called "doubly labelled water" which enabled us to estimate how many calories she was really consuming. When we totted up her diary it came to 1500 calories. The doubly labelled water technique suggested she was consuming far more than that. Before you tut-tut, it's easily done.

The other bit of tech worth investing in is some way of tracking how many steps you do. This could be an app, a pedometer or a fitbit. You need to record how many steps you do over a typical week before you start on the diet. It's likely to be around 5000. Whatever it is, I want you to write it down, and then aim to increase the number of steps you take by around 10% a week for the course of the diet. By the end I would hope you would be doing at least 10,000 steps, maybe more. I'll explain later why 10,000 steps is such an important figure.

Measure your pulse, weight and waist

Find a quiet moment and measure your pulse. You will find it throbbing away on your wrist, just outside the outermost tendon. Your pulse is a measure of your overall fitness. Measure it a few times, then write down the average score. I'd expect to see it improve over the coming few weeks.

Next I want you to weigh yourself. So, up to the bathroom and on to the digital scales. With this figure, and your height, you can calculate your BMI. See the appendix at the back of the book for how to do this, or go to our website thebloodsugardiet.com, which will do it automatically for you.

While you are in the bathroom, I want you to whip out a tape measure and measure your waist size. Honestly. There is no point in trying to hold everything in. You measure your waist size by going around your belly button; do not rely on your trouser size. Men typically underestimate their waist size by about 2–3in.

Why is waist size important? Because it is an indirect measure of your visceral fat and one of the best predictors we have of future health. As I've pointed out before, fat in and around the abdomen is dangerous even if you are not otherwise obviously overweight.

Ideally your waist should be less than half your height (so if you are six feet tall your waist should be less than 36in).

According to a recent survey of more than 32,000

American men and women,[39] waist sizes in the US are expanding at a frightening rate. Between 2009 and 2011 the average American male's waist grew from 39 to nearly 40in; the average woman's belly expanded even more, from 36 to 38in.

This is a whopping 12in more than average waist sizes in the 1950s. Marilyn Monroe, who had a 22in waist, was not exceptional for her time. Frank Hu, Professor of Nutrition and Epidemiology at the Harvard School of Public Health, thinks that high-sugar diets and increased stress hormones may be largely responsible.

So that's your pulse, weight and waist measured and noted down. And while you're at it, take some selfies. Or preferably get a friend to take photos of you. Keep this somewhere safe so you can compare the outward changes of having done this diet. I predict that you will want to show people the "before" and "after".

Measure your fasting glucose
This is a finger prick test you can do yourself (you can buy reliable digital blood sugar monitoring kits at chemists and online) or you may prefer to ask your doctor to do it. It should be done in the fasting state, i.e. first thing in the morning, before breakfast, when you have not eaten for at least eight hours. If it comes back abnormal you will need to repeat it and do further tests.

Normal range: 3.9 to 5.5mmol/l (70 to 100mg/dl)
Prediabetes: 5.6 to 7.0mmol/l (101 to 125mg/dl)
Diabetic: more than 7.0mmol/l (125mg/dl)

There is disagreement about exactly where "normal" ends and prediabetes begins. The figures above are from the American Diabetes Association. The WHO (World Health Organisation) says "normal" is under 6.1mmol/l (110mg/dl), while NICE (National Institute of Clinical Excellence) recommends you keep below 5.9mmol/l (106mg/dl).

Other routine tests you should ask your doctor about include HbA1C, an FBC (full blood count), U&Es (urea and electrolytes), liver function tests (including Gamma GT, a good measure of how healthy your liver is), cholesterol and blood lipid profile.

It would be more unusual to get your insulin levels measured, but if you do your doctor will be able to calculate how insulin-resistant you are. I have included more details on all these in the appendix.

Specialist scanning tests
The following tests are not routine but they are revealing and can be highly motivating:

1. Dual-energy X-ray absorptiometry or DXA scan.
    This is used to measure visceral fat. By doing a DXA

at the start, four weeks in and at the end, you can track changes as you go along. It is more expensive but also more reliable than simply weighing yourself. Sticking DXA images to your fridge door will remind you why you are doing this.

2. Liver ultrasound scan. Like the Gamma GT blood test, this is a way of assessing the health of your liver. It will give you an estimate of how much fat you have in it.

3. Magnetic Resonance Imaging (MRI). This is the most accurate way of measuring liver and pancreatic fat, but it is time-consuming and expensive. If you want to see an MRI of my body when I was 20lb heavier and a TOFI (Thin on the Outside, Fat Inside), then go to thebloodsugardiet.com. All that white stuff smothering my liver and pancreas is fat. Be warned. It's not pretty.

Clear out your cupboards – "kitchen hygiene"

Don't keep food you want to avoid eating in the house. It might sound obvious but if sugary snacks are anywhere to hand, unless you have superhuman willpower, there will come a time when you will eat them. My daughter has never forgiven me for eating her Easter egg when she was 10. It was sitting there, in full view. I couldn't resist taking a bite. Then another. Then it was all gone.

If you have children and feel you have to have sweet or savoury treats in the house it's a bit more difficult. If you are fortunate enough to have a partner who isn't a carb addict, get them to keep the treats in a locked cupboard. I'm not kidding. I sometimes have a bit of chocolate after a meal, but I get my wife to hide the bar; otherwise I would eat the whole lot. The safest course of action is to give it all away. The junk has to go. It will, however, leave space for healthier foods…

Write down your goals

When you are in the thick of a new eating regime, you will inevitably have moments of doubt or forget why you are putting yourself through it. So, before you start, jot down all the reasons why you want to get your blood sugar under control. Keep it with you. Make it into your screen saver. Read this list whenever you feel yourself weakening. Make the reasons as specific as you can.

Remember, you have really good reasons – what psychologists call "a driver" – to change. This isn't about vanity (though you will almost certainly look better). It isn't about what size your jeans are (though you should drop several sizes). It's about getting healthy. It's about getting your life back.

One of the goals you absolutely have to write down is how much weight you plan to lose. Any amount will help, particularly if you are in the prediabetes phase, but to properly reverse type 2 diabetes you will probably need to lose 10–15% of your current body weight. I lost 20lb, which was 11% of my body weight, and that for me did the trick. If your original BMI is over 40, then you may need to lose more.

As I've mentioned before, we all have different fat thresholds – that is, the weight at which type 2 diabetes is reversed – so it is important to know what's happening to your blood sugar while doing the diet, which is why I suggest you invest in that digital blood sugar monitor…

Find a diet buddy

Being part of a group – even if it's just you and one friend – will significantly improve your chances of success.

Once you've decided that you want to go on this diet then tell your friends and family all about it. They may know someone else who wants to do it with you. The fact that you are making a public commitment also means you are more likely to stick to it.

When should I start?

The sooner the better. That said, you should find a period in your life when you know you can clear at least six weeks to focus on losing weight. It's fine to keep working. Keeping busy will actually help. But make sure your work colleagues are on board and not dumping doughnuts on your desk to "cheer you up". Likewise, you don't want your 50th birthday or your friend's wedding to derail you, but don't look for excuses not to start.

Once you've talked to your doctor, done your tests, cleared the junk food out of your cupboards, taped your goals to the fridge and found a dieting buddy, it's time to get going.

"Going on this diet is like preparing for an expedition."

When Paul starts craving a breakfast muffin with eggs and bacon and brown sauce, he does something that might horrify you (it certainly horrifies him): he goes online and looks up pictures of feet just before they are to be amputated. This is a man who is taking it seriously. Very seriously.

Paul – who describes himself as "a real foodie. Shopping, cooking, consuming food – it's all a great pleasure to me" – asked his doctor to give him three months' grace to turn round his type 2 diagnosis.

Soon after starting the diet he began doing the training sessions I detail in this book – a workout for muscle building and an aerobic routine. He supplemented this routine with long walks and bicycle rides. Every morning he measured his blood sugars and wrote the results down in a book.

His advice? "It is like preparing for an expedition. You can't do it half-heartedly. You have to commit. It is like flicking a switch – you just have to think to yourself, 'I am not going to do anything that jeopardises this.'"

He was 171lb (78kg) when he was diagnosed. Like 35% of type 2 diabetics, his BMI was within the healthy range.

However, he knew he was at risk: his mother is diabetic and when he puts on weight it settles around his middle – a clear danger sign. "I was walking around with my head in the sand," he says. "I kept putting off addressing it."

Then two years ago his wife died from breast cancer (an emotional upheaval, as we have seen, is often part of the story). He started drinking more – and his weight crept up. Going on the diet was, in a way, a sign that it was time for a new chapter in his life to begin.

"It's a line in the sand. It has been very positive. It means that I want to take care of myself again. It means I have climbed out of a trough of despond and I am looking after myself. It's significant. A way of taking control again in a way that I had lost. To feel that I can – and I want – to do this is empowering."

Chapter seven

THE DIET IN PRACTICE

You have decided to go for it. You have talked to your doctor, cleared your cupboards and done some tests. As you will soon discover, the BSD isn't quite as tough as you may fear. Yes, you are going to be living on 800 calories a day for the next few weeks, but your body should adapt reasonably quickly. There is one final decision to make: do you want to do the diet entirely with real food, or do you want to do it in part with commercial meal-replacement diet shakes?

Two ways to go

In Professor Taylor's studies, largely for reasons of convenience, the subjects were asked to lose weight by drinking commercial meal-replacement diet shakes for the whole eight weeks, supplemented with some non-starchy vegetables. If you are running a scientific study, using diet shakes is not only convenient but also an easier way to keep close tabs on just how many calories people are actually consuming. But others have done it very successfully on real food. It's a personal decision. You have to decide which suits you best.

Meal-replacement shakes

If you decide to start with meal-replacement diet shakes, you should aim to consume around 600 calories per day in shakes, plus 200 calories in non-starchy vegetables. You will need that extra fibre from the vegetables (plus lots of water) to stop yourself getting constipated. We have provided some 200-calorie recipes – vegetable dishes and soups – in the recipe section later in the book.

The advantages of reputable meal-replacement diet shakes is that you know you are getting a balance of the right nutrients and you don't have to think about food. The disadvantage is that none of the commercial shakes I've tried so far have been particularly pleasant. I imagine that in time they would get boring.

I also think it is important, while you are on the diet, to learn how to cook proper, healthy, delicious meals. This will prepare you for life after the diet. A reasonable compromise might be to start with the shakes, get settled in, then after you have been on the diet for, say, two weeks switch to eating mostly real food.

Real food

Doing the diet with real food is slightly harder because you have to make sure that you are getting the right amount of protein, fat, vitamins, etc. That is why I asked Dr Sarah Schenker, one of the UK's leading dieticians, to provide a range of simple, nutritious recipes, as well as a detailed and balanced dietary plan (see pages 255-59).

The principle behind the recipes is Mediterranean-style, low-carb eating. They are packed with nutrients and decent amounts of fats and proteins; they are flavoursome and varied so there is less chance that your taste buds will get bored and start craving the bad stuff.

If you want to do your own thing and make up your own Med-style, low-carb recipes, then do make sure that you are getting a varied diet with adequate amounts of the right nutrients. You may want to take a daily multivitamin pill to be on the safe side. I think one of the other main advantages of doing this diet with real food is that this will retrain your taste buds. You may be someone who is not currently particularly fond of vegetables, but when you are on a low-calorie diet they will taste delicious! Remember, you are resetting your body not just for the next few months, but hopefully for good.

Q & A

What does 800 calories look like?
More than you might think (check out the picture section

138

in this book where seven days × 800 cals are laid out for you) – but less than you're used to. The key to this diet is that every single mouthful packs a punch. And it scores high on what dieticians call the satiety factor – the feeling of fullness after eating that suppresses the urge to eat between meals. You should feel satisfied by smaller portions and won't stay forever hungry and preoccupied by food. As you watch the weight fall off you will get a lot of positive reinforcement to keep you going.

Why 800 calories? Why not eat more, or less...

If you have problems with blood sugar and want to regain your health, then you need to lose fat, particularly abdominal fat. It doesn't really matter how quickly or slowly you do it; it's just that you may find it easier to lose it fast. Losing weight fast, if it's done properly, is motivating. Eight hundred calories is low, as diets go, but not super low.

There are carbohydrates in this diet, yet you say I shouldn't eat them

There are some carbohydrates in the menus provided – but the right sort. As you will know by now, starchy carbohydrates are essentially concentrated sugars and are disruptive to blood sugar. You will find recipes here that include jumbo oats, and even brown rice – but in small quantities. It's a taste, not a main component of the meal. These carbohydrates are the slow-burn kind, meaning they take time and energy to digest, which means you'll feel less hungry.

So what's going to keep me feeling full up?

Fat and protein keep you feeling fuller for longer. The standard recommendations for protein are around 45g a day for a woman, and 55g per day for a man. Good proteins to eat include eggs, fish, chicken, pork, prawns and tofu. Nuts, seeds and pulses are packed full of protein too.

Is this a low-fat diet?

No – because, as I explained earlier, fat isn't the bad guy that it was once made out to be. It includes plenty of fish, a judicious amount of animal fat from meat, and plenty of plant fat (i.e. from nuts, seeds, olive oil, avocados), as well as yoghurt (unsugared). On the other hand, to lose weight fast you have to cut down on calories, so you won't find handfuls of cheese in the recipes (although there is a little strong-tasting holiday-recalling feta here and there.)

Is snacking on fruit OK?

Fruit contains far more sugar than vegetables. There is some fruit in this diet but it is rationed and used as an ingredient rather than an excuse to eat between meals. If you're looking for something to chop up and stir through yoghurt, go for deep-coloured blueberries, blackcurrants, cherries or strawberries. But limit your intake of tropical fruit, which tends to be higher in sugar. And steer clear of dates. Even at Christmas. Eating two dates has the same effect on your blood sugar as eating two large punnets of strawberries.

In that case – are some vegetables better than others?

Absolutely. Some are starchier than others, which means they will affect your blood sugar. Leafy green vegetables like broccoli, spinach, cabbage, lettuce, kale, chard and cauliflower are rich in vitamin C and fibre and very low in sugar and starch, so tuck in. Ditto tomatoes, cucumbers and peppers. It gets more complicated with root vegetables – potatoes, parsnips, swedes – these are quite high in starch so should be treated with more caution.

Do I have to eat breakfast?

It's a myth that everyone has to eat breakfast. I love it, but some people don't. In the recipe section there are some brilliant weekend brunch dishes, which take a bit longer to cook and are more calorific, but because you will be eating two meals on those days you can get away with it. There is the added advantage that you will have fasted for about 14 hours overnight.

What's so good about nuts?

Nuts have traditionally had a bad rap because they are oily and high in calories. However, you will find some nuts in the recipes because they are high in protein and fibre. They are satiating and do not cause much upsurge in blood sugar levels. They are an important component of the Mediterranean diet.

What about seeds?

Seeds may be tiny, but they're packed with nutrients like protein, fibre, iron, vitamins and omega-3 fatty acids. Whether you choose chia seeds or flax, pumpkin seeds or hemp – sprinkle them in your salads, use them to make green vegetables more interesting, or stir them through yoghurt. They will help you to feel fuller for longer. What's not to like?

Can I drink alcohol?

When you are on the diet, preferably not. If you have to, then stick to small amounts of spirits. Alcohol is highly calorific. A pint of beer contains around 180 calories. Ditto a large glass of wine. Red wine is lower in sugar than white, but the calories still add up. Five glasses of wine a week amounts to 900 calories, the same as four doughnuts. Alcohol will also increase fat storage and inflammation in the liver, increasing the insulin resistance that promotes weight gain and diabetes. A number of people I have talked to while researching this book can date their blood sugar problems back to consuming too much booze.

What if I'm a prediabetic, not yet a type 2?

If, after doing the tests, you have discovered that you are

Day One

Breakfast: Blueberry and green tea shake
Lunch: Pepper with jewelled feta
Dinner: Aubergine with lamb and pomegranate
Calories: 810

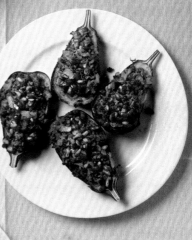

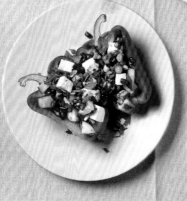

Day Two

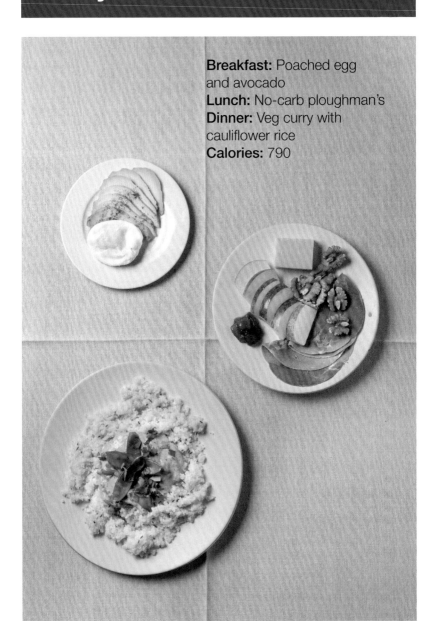

Breakfast: Poached egg and avocado
Lunch: No-carb ploughman's
Dinner: Veg curry with cauliflower rice
Calories: 790

Day Three

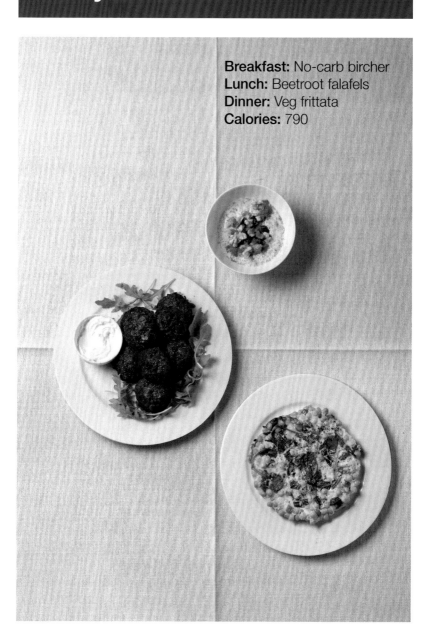

Breakfast: No-carb bircher
Lunch: Beetroot falafels
Dinner: Veg frittata
Calories: 790

Breakfast: Portobello 'toast' with goat's cheese and pine nuts
Lunch: Sardine dip
Dinner: Foil-steamed fish
Calories: 840

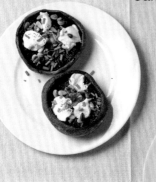
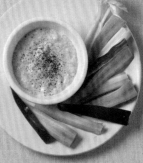
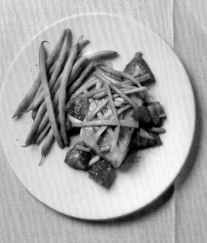

Day Five

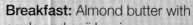

Breakfast: Almond butter with apple and goji berries
Lunch: Warm halloumi salad
Dinner: Spicy chicken with lentils
Calories: 860

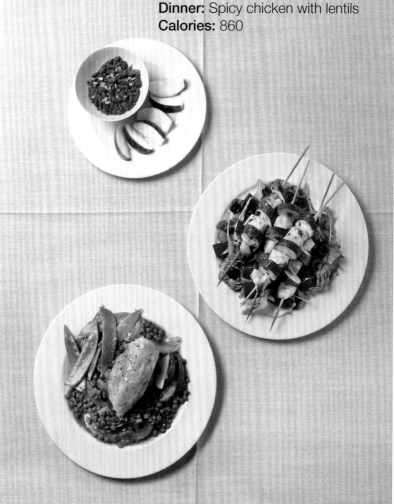

Day Six

Brunch: Cheesy baked beans
Dinner: Steak with crème fraîche and peppercorn sauce
Calories: 770

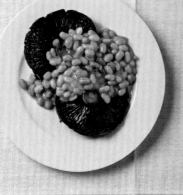

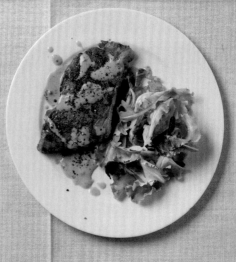

Day Seven

Brunch: Poached egg and salmon stack
Dinner: Harissa chicken
Calories: 740

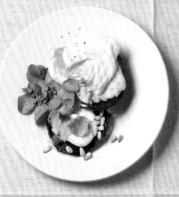

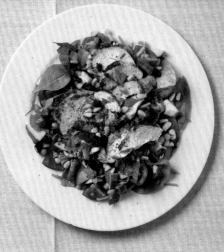

Instant Soups

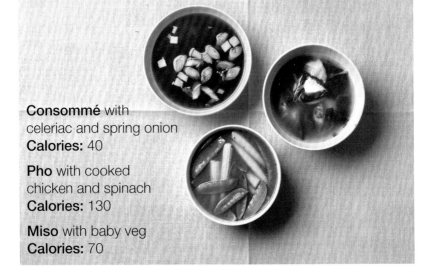

Consommé with celeriac and spring onion
Calories: 40

Pho with cooked chicken and spinach
Calories: 130

Miso with baby veg
Calories: 70

Blood Sugar Diet **favourite ingredients**

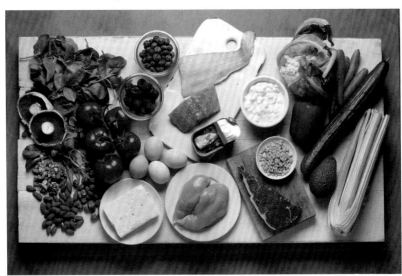

prediabetic and overweight rather than fully diabetic, you could certainly try doing the diet until you've got your blood sugars back to normal levels. There is good evidence that losing weight and maintaining an exercise programme will significantly reduce your risk of progressing from prediabetes to diabetes. In a trial run by the National Institutes of Health in the US,[40] which recruited over 3000 people with prediabetes, they found that 7% weight loss combined with an exercise regime cut the participants' risk of developing diabetes by 58% over the next five years. For more on the Diabetes Prevention Program visit http://www.cdc.gov/diabetes/prevention/about.htm

Diet timeline:
what to do and what to expect

The first two weeks

Once you've started you will find that you begin to lose weight, fast. Some of it will be fat but initially you will also be passing a lot of urine. It is essential that you drink at least 2–3 litres of calorie-free fluid a day or you will become constipated and get headaches. What you drink is up to you, as long as it doesn't contain calories. It could be ordinary tap water. If you are not keen on plain water, try flavouring it with a squeeze of lemon or lime, or fresh mint and cucumber. I love fizzy water with lots of ice and lemon. Or plenty of fruit tea and the occasional coffee (but only a splash of milk). Some people like hot water, and oddly enough there is evidence that heat alone can soothe hunger. Zero-calorie fizzy drinks if you must. But not fruit juice or smoothies.

The first two weeks are likely to be the toughest, as your body adapts to fewer calories, but this should in turn lead to some dramatic changes. To give you a flavour of what you are likely to experience and the sort of changes you can expect, I asked a friend of mine, Dick, who was about to start the diet, to keep a detailed diary.

"It was how to eat less – but eat better."

Dick is a foodie. Nothing wrong with that but he was eating big portions and drinking too much. "I am not a binge drinker," he told me, "but six o'clock used to be time for the first gin and tonic. And I don't mean a small one. Then most of a bottle of wine. Followed by a few whiskies." Dick may have been exaggerating – but only a little.

Even his non-alcoholic drinks were calorific. He would start each day with four sugars in his mug of tea.

He was overweight at 215lb (97.5kg) and with

a 42in waist. He was beginning to look not only paunchy, but also uncharacteristically grey and ill. Shortly after being diagnosed as a diabetic he contacted me for advice. We agreed that he would aim to lose 30lb (around 15% of his body weight) and get his blood sugars (which were over 9mmol/l) back down to normal within eight weeks. He also wanted to lose 6in from his waist. He had a good-natured bet with his doctor, who said he wouldn't do it.

Over the first few weeks he managed not only to surprise his doctor, but also to debunk every myth about rapid weight loss.

He didn't feel deprived
On Day 3 of the diet he wrote in his diary, "Still feeling fine. Weird. Not light-headed 'weird'. Weird as in 'Everyone told me this wouldn't be possible and I'd be desperate enough to eat the dog, but that is so not the case.'"

By then his fasting glucose was already down 30% and when he stood on the scales he found that he had lost over 7lb (3kg). In three days. As he wrote, "I know this will slow down but it's very motivating."

He did the cooking for himself and his wife, Alison. His meals were delicious: sea bass fillet with leafy greens, smoked kipper fillets with a poached egg, lemon sole with vegetables, tray-bake chicken with red peppers, tomatoes and onion. He put aside the bread, pasta and potatoes.

He set himself a challenge – "The goal wasn't to worry about how I can survive on only 800 calories. It was 'How can I make those 800 calories really tasty and fulfilling?' It was how to eat less – but eat better."

He didn't feel miserable

He lost almost 10lb (4.5kg) in the first seven days. By Day 9 his blood sugar levels had fallen to normal. His delight is clear – "Yes!! First result under the diabetes threshold!! For today I am not diabetic."

Two days later the reading was down again. He wrote, "Hello pancreas!"

He was hugely encouraged to see that it was all happening so rapidly. "You are dropping so fast. And it happens almost immediately." The fact that he was in control, doing something about his health, also spurred him on – "Just recently, life hadn't been the success it has always been in the past. This turned that feeling around for me."

He maintained both his work and his social life. He kept on track by telling people what he was doing, avoiding refined carbohydrates, planning ahead, making sensible food choices. Dick would be the first to agree – it wasn't rocket science.

He started to walk more. Not just by going for actual walks but also by playing several rounds of golf a week. This added up to around 4000 extra steps a day.

The hunger wasn't hard to deal with
Dick used MyFitnessApp, which scanned and measured everything he ate (and produced a report of calories and food contents) and took some of the emotion out of what he was eating – or, rather, not eating. He realised that the times when he thought he was hungry, it was often merely a craving and if he did something else – walk the dog, for instance – the feeling would pass. Not being able to drink alcohol was, admittedly, trickier. After the first week he began to sneak in the odd whisky. He still lost weight.

It wasn't all plain sailing. There were days when his sugar levels nudged upwards but he didn't let these derail him. They were lapses, not relapses. The following day, helped by keeping the diary which kept him mindful of what he was doing, he got back on track.

It took Dick 34 days to see his blood sugar results stabilise in the normal range and two months to get down to 186lb (84kg).

That was a year ago, and he maintains his weight loss by continuing to be active and eating a low carb diet. His blood sugars are still in the normal range. I haven't seen him looking so well for a long time. Occasionally he indulges in bread, but only a single slice, or small portions of sweet potatoes. When he does this he sees his blood sugar levels rise, so he's decided it's simply not worth doing it that often.

Reasons why he succeeded?

- He was motivated
- He really believed the theory behind this rapid diet – it made sense to him
- He takes great pleasure in proving people wrong
- Especially his doctor – who hasn't yet paid out on their bet
- His wife, Alison, is a huge support

After the first two weeks

Dick managed to lose 15lb (7kg) in his first two weeks on the diet and as his weight dropped his blood sugar levels also fell. But, though he had lost fat from his liver, his pancreas was still clogged. It was important he keep going, lose more inches round his waist. If he had stopped the diet at two weeks his blood sugars would probably have gone back up again.

Not everyone needs to do the full eight weeks. If you

are prediabetic or slim to begin with (see Richard's story, below), then two weeks may be long enough for you to reach your goal – in which case, you can move on to the BSD way of life (see page 155).

Most overweight diabetics, however, will probably need to press on. Hopefully, you will not only have been following the weight loss regime but also boosting your activity and mindfulness (see chapters eight and nine). The important thing is how you are feeling – are you coping? Here are a few questions to ask yourself:

1. Are you losing weight at a steady pace? By the end of Week 2 it may have slowed but it should still be rapid.
2. Is your appetite under better control? Most people report feeling less hungry by the end of Week 2.
3. Are your blood sugar levels coming down or are they still all over the place?
4. Are you sleeping? If not, you may wish to eat your main meal a bit later.
5. Are you getting constipated? If so I would recommend not only drinking more fluids but also adding more fibre-rich food, i.e. non-starchy vegetables.
6. Are you coping emotionally? You may feel more irritable but I would be concerned about a prolonged drop in mood.
7. Are you managing to stick with the diet most of the time?

If the answer is "no" to more than two of these questions, this may not be the right diet for you. Rather than give up I recommend you try what I call the 5:2 approach, cutting your calories down to 800 for two days, and staying on a low-carb Mediterranean-style eating plan for the rest of the week. It will be slower but as long as you lose the weight it should still be effective. See page 162 for more details.

The reason for having a review after two weeks is that it gives you long enough to get into the swing of things. Hopefully you are feeling in control, slimmer, energised. But I also want to be sure that you are not pushing yourself too hard. Diets can be tough even if you are in perfect health. If you are a diabetic there are added pitfalls.

I was recently contacted by John, an American in his early fifties. John has always been really fit and active. Earlier this year he began to feel tired and very thirsty all the time. So he went to his doctor, had a blood test, and discovered that his blood sugars were sky high.

His doctor thought, largely because of his age, that John must be a type 2 diabetic. Yet he was slim, and a DXA scan showed he had hardly any visceral fat. None-the-less John wanted to see if a very low-calorie diet would help. It didn't.

After two weeks he had lost weight but he didn't feel good and his blood sugars were still out of control, even on medication. He went back to his doctor, who decided he was probably not a type 2, after all, but a late onset type 1 diabetic.

Most type 1 diabetics develop the condition as children or in early adulthood, but some do so much later in life. John's blood sugar problems were not caused by too much liver fat but because his pancreas had been damaged by his own immune system. He is now managing his blood sugar levels with medication and a lowish-carb diet.

So, John is a cautionary tale. Richard, on the other hand, is an example of just how effective rapid weight loss can be if your problem really is too much visceral fat.

> *"At work they started calling me*
> *'The Disappearing Man'."*

We all have different tipping points, and there can be quite wide variations between the points at which people start to see big improvements in their blood sugar control. Richard Doughty managed to get his blood sugar under control in 11 days. Less time than an average family's summer holiday.

How did the 59-year-old journalist do it? He chose a time when his wife was away in South Africa – "I didn't want her to worry. And she might think that I was being a bit daft" – and when he didn't have any big family events in the diary. "There were about five months of umming and ahhing and finding a time when I knew I would be able to stick to it."

At the same time he was absolutely determined. "It was such a shock, getting the diagnosis. But I can be very single-minded."

He made sure he carried on his life in just the same way as before (albeit with lots of healthy soups and feeling the cold despite it being July). He went to work. He even played cricket.

What were the hardest things about the diet?

Being told he looked too thin! Because Doughty is one of those skinny-fat people I mentioned earlier, a TOFI – no one was more surprised than he was to discover his blood sugar status. When he started losing weight people told him he was too scrawny. "At work they started calling me 'The Disappearing Man'," he says. "But better looking thin than missing a foot."

He lost 9lb (4kg) in 11 days – by which time his blood sugars had returned to normal. He waited two months before he saw his doctor again. His blood sugar levels were still comfortably below the diabetes mark. He has since had regular tests and each time the results are fine. When he talks about the turnaround you can still hear the delight in his voice. He dieted his way back to non-diabetes in less time than it takes for a tennis player to win Wimbledon.

The four-week review

The next key moment in your dieting odyssey will be the four-week review. By now you are halfway through the diet and hopefully things are going well. You will have lost a lot of weight, with much of it coming off your waist. Your blood sugars will be starting to stabilise at close to normal levels. Your sugar cravings should be much reduced.

Retake our Carbs Craving Quiz and see how you are doing.

Ideally, at the four-week mark, you should revisit your doctor to repeat blood tests and scans, if you did them before you started the diet.

Just as with the two-week review, by the end of four weeks some will have reached their goals, in which case they should celebrate and move on to the maintenance phase (see page 155). Others may be finding it hard going. But don't give up. Moving to a 5:2 approach or going straight on to the maintenance programme are viable options.

So, what changes can you realistically expect to see in your weight and blood sugars by the end of four weeks?

Well, in Professor Taylor's original study[41] his volunteers, who started out at over 200lb (90.5kg), lost an average of 22lb (10kg) by the end of four weeks, most of it fat. They also lost nearly 3in round the waist. Other changes that happened by four weeks included:

Fasting glucose	down from 9.2 to 5.7 mmol/l
Fasting insulin	down from 151 to 57 pmol/l
Gamma GT (liver test)	down from 62 to 25 U/1

Again, however, a note of caution. As I mentioned earlier, when Professor Taylor did a follow-up study,[42] this time with people who were older and had been diabetic for much longer, the results were mixed.

Those who had been diabetic for less than five years did really well. But those who'd been diabetic for more than eight years and were on lots of medication were less likely to see rapid improvements in their blood sugar levels.

That said, everyone reported feeling better, sleeping better and being more active. Blood pressure and cholesterol levels also improved across the board.

At the end of eight weeks

By the end of the 8-week diet, if not before, you will see some big changes in your body shape and biochemistry. You should be sleeping better, and feeling a real sense of achievement. Perhaps you need to buy some new trousers. Maybe you stop and look in mirrors to admire the difference. So, pull out that old photo. Take a new one. Post them on Facebook or Twitter.

By the end of eight weeks most people will have

reached their targets, but some won't. Perhaps you have more weight to lose, maybe your blood sugars or HbA1C results have not improved as much as you would have hoped. If you feel you are heading in the right direction, but are just not quite there yet, I suggest that rather than continue of eating 800 calories every day, you move to the more flexible 5:2 approach (see page 162).

The end of the diet is also a good time to visit your doctor, redo the tests, print off the graphs if you have tracked your progress and celebrate what you have done with family and friends.

Getting this far is a real achievement, but you don't want to undo all the good work by going back to living the way you used to. Your main preoccupation now should be, "How am I going to stay in this shape for the rest of my life?"

The BSD Way of Life

As I'm sure you know, many people who go on a diet end up putting on some, if not most, of the weight they have so painfully lost. But this is not inevitable. The main thing you have to do is create a lifestyle you can stick to. If this involves avoiding all your favourite foods and running 20 miles a day then it will fail. Be realistic.

Don't despair. Lots of others have lost weight and kept it off. I lost 22lb (10kg) three years ago and occasionally I put a couple of pounds back on. But I find I can rapidly lose it again.

I'm sure the main reason I've succeeded in keeping off the weight is that I've gone from gorging on sugary carbs to following a Med-style eating plan. That, along with increased activity and practising mindfulness (see chapter nine), has helped me keep diabetes at bay.

The following are a few other things I've found useful and which are now a way of life for me. They are based on numerous conversations with diet experts:

- **We try to sit down at the kitchen table for every meal.** If you eat on the run or in front of the TV you will eat badly and go on eating well beyond the point when you would normally feel full. A striking example of this was when researchers from the University of Southern California gave people going into a cinema buckets of stale popcorn.[43] The people who normally eat popcorn at a cinema wolfed it down, despite the fact it tasted terrible. This demonstrates how little attention we pay to what we are eating when we are distracted.

- **I try to eat slowly.** It takes time for the food you eat to reach the parts of your small intestine where cells release a hormone,

PYY, that tells your brain, "I'm full". That's why if you eat slowly you will eat less. I regularly put my knife and fork down for a while and try to wait 30 seconds or so before picking them up again. I also now leave food on my plate when I am no longer hungry. This goes against everything I was taught when growing up.

- **I avoid "diet" products** as they are highly processed and often contain sugar and/or sweeteners (which may not switch off hunger signals).

- **I drink soup a lot.** It is satiating, cheap and practical. We make big quantities, often out of left-over veg, and keep the unused stuff in the freezer.

- **Don't drink lots of alcohol.** Alcohol contains plenty of calories and makes you disinhibited, so you are more likely to snack. I have switched to drinking red wine and try to drink only when I am eating. I also leave the bottle on the other side of the room because I know that I am less likely to fill my glass regularly if I have to get up. For similar reasons we leave the salt in the cupboard rather than on the table, and any remaining food gets left on the cooker. I am less likely to help myself to more if I have to cross the room.

- **Keep tempting foods out of the house or out of sight.** The kids sometimes sneak chocolate and biscuits in, but know better than to leave them anywhere they can be spotted. In a fascinating study Cornell University researchers went round houses in Syracuse, New York, taking photos of people's kitchens. They found they could predict a family's weight by the foods left out on the surface. If breakfast cereals, for example, were visible, the inhabitants were, on average, 21lb heavier than people in households where the cereals were put away. Breakfast cereals have a reputation for being healthy. They aren't.[44]

- **Don't keep your cupboards empty.** If there's no food in the house you will probably order a takeaway. Make sure there's plenty of food around like nuts, yoghurt and eggs. Keep the fridge stocked with vegetable crudités, such as sticks of carrots, green peppers or tomatoes, perhaps with some salsa or hummus, for moments when you just have to snack. Put them at eye level in the fridge. Anything unhealthily calorific needs to be covered up and stored in the bottom of the fridge where you are less likely to see it. My weakness is toast. I did suggest to my wife we throw the toaster out (on the grounds that I would rarely bother to use the grill) but she refused. Instead, I keep unsalted nuts by the toaster, so when I am tempted to snack on toast and marmalade I eat nuts instead. Mostly.

- **I weigh myself several times a week.** Scales can be extraordinarily fickle; sometimes my weight seems to go up and down like a yo-yo. There is a widely held belief that you shouldn't weigh yourself more than once a week. Yet a recent study suggests more is better. In this particular trial,[45] they followed 40 people attending a health promotion programme. Some weighed themselves daily, others weekly, monthly or hardly at all. The more often people weighed themselves the more weight they lost.

- **Wear a belt.** One of the surest ways of telling that you are putting on unhealthy fat is noticing when your belt starts to feel tight again.

- **When we go out for a meal** I make sure the waiters never leave the bread basket on the table, or I would just help myself. I stick to one course, with lots of vegetables instead of rice or potatoes. I rarely have a dessert and when I do I always share it with someone else. Research shows that a small amount of something sticky and tasty is just as satisfying as eating a large portion.

- **I try not to go shopping on an empty stomach** and aim to fill half the basket, at least, with healthy stuff. When I pick up a cake, I always look at the label. The huge number of calories and vast amounts of sugar normally make me put it back on the shelf. I used to kid myself that if I bought cake or a packet or biscuits I would eat only a small amount. I know that's not true. For the same reason I never buy large bars of chocolate, however much of a bargain they seem.

- **I always take the stairs** and I normally try to run up them. I think it is sad how many people stand on escalators when they could be burning a few extra calories walking up them.

- **When I get cravings for something sweet** I buy sugar-free chewing gum. Cravings are all about imagining the tastes and textures of the forbidden food. It is almost impossible to think about the taste of chocolate when you are munching on gum.

- **We got a dog**, Tari, and she barks loudly if we don't take her for a walk at least once a day. Not the most practical tip if you live in the city or prefer cats.

- **Keep busy.** Take up a new hobby that will keep your body and mind active. I took up Latin American dancing when I was fasting. It got my heart going and was mentally challenging.

- **I acknowledge "three good things".** This is based on an idea devised by American psychologist Professor Martin Seligman. All you do, at the end of the day, is think of and/ or write down three things that went well that day and why they went well. It doesn't have to be anything major; perhaps someone complimented you, or you watched a beautiful sunset. The point is that it focuses your attention on the positive. It is a good way to lift your mood and bolster resilience.

- **Most weeks I try to fast.** I have one day when I try to go at least 12 hours without food. I do this by having breakfast, skipping lunch and having a light evening meal. There are health benefits from short periods of fasting. Fasting also reminds me that I can control hunger and that it doesn't control me.

The less intensive BSD – going 5:2

We are all different. Many people – including those who have provided the case studies for this book – find 800 calories a day surprisingly easy and just keep going. It does work well on people who are motivated, and I hope that is how it works out for you.

But no one diet is going to suit everyone. If you begin the diet and really don't feel well on it, or you find 800 calories a day, every day, either too tough or too inconvenient to stick to for the full eight weeks, then I would recommend the 5:2 approach as a gentler alternative.

The 5:2 approach is very simple. For five days of the week you don't calorie-count but simply go on the low-carb Mediterranean diet I described earlier. Then, for two days a week, you cut down your calories to 800 a day using the menus in this book. You can do this on any two days of the week that suit you, but it is best to be consistent so you get into a pattern. Try consecutive days, such as Monday and Tuesday. Or you may prefer to split your days, Monday and Thursday. Whatever works for you.

You won't lose weight as fast as you would if you stuck to 800 calories a day, but it can be more effective than conventional dieting. Studies suggest the 5:2 approach is easier to stick to; you lose fat (rather than muscle) faster and you see bigger improvements in your insulin sensitivity.[46]

I've written extensively about the health and weight loss benefits of the 5:2 "intermittent fasting" diet elsewhere (*The Fast Diet*; thefastdiet.co.uk).

In the original version of the Fast Diet, I recommended men stick to 600 calories a day, and women to 500, twice a week. Going up to 800 calories is unlikely to make that much of a difference, particularly if you go low-carb on the other five days.

The 5:2 diet was how I reversed my own diabetes, and since I wrote that book I have had many emails from people who are now "former diabetics", including one from Leo, who had been a type 2 diabetic for 12 years.

Despite being on medication, Leo's blood sugars were getting so bad that in 2012 his doctor told him he needed to start on insulin injections. Instead, Leo did my 5:2 diet, lost 44lb (20kg) in three months, and became drug-free. Three years later he has put on a few pounds but his blood sugars remain fine.

What should I do about check-ups?

If you were prediabetic and you have a personal blood glucose monitor, I would recommend, at least initially, that you do monthly fasting blood sugar checks, just to make sure you are keeping on track. You also need to have yearly blood sugar checks through your doctor. If you go back to your previous lifestyle and activity, then, over time, you are at risk of becoming prediabetic again.

If you were a type 2 diabetic, you will need to go on having regular diabetic check-ups with your doctor. Usually this will be at least yearly. If your blood sugar levels remain in the normal range, your doctor may be happy for you to have these checks less often. But don't just stop going for reviews as it is important to make sure your kidneys, eyes, feet, cardiovascular system and other organs have not been affected.

What should I do if things start going in the wrong direction?

First of all, review your diet: are you slipping in more of the high-GI, simple carbohydrates than you need? Have your portions got bigger? If you are serious about wanting to stay healthy, you will have to act. This may involve simply cutting out the extra treats you have allowed yourself, or adding in a few weeks of intermittent fasting (see the BSD 5:2 option above). Some people make the 5:2 approach their maintenance programme, or they go for a 6:1 approach (sticking to 800 calories for one day out of seven). Research shows that even if you do it only one day a week you can get the metabolic benefits of fasting, such as improved insulin sensitivity.

Next, review your exercise and activity levels: are you still taking the stairs, doing a regular walk, fitting in some resistance exercises (see next chapter)?

Are you going through a period of disruption and stress in your life? If so, the raised cortisol can upset your blood sugars. Chapter nine is all about techniques for de-stressing and reducing comfort eating.

Finally, don't despair or give up. Putting on a bit of weight after you have stopped dieting is normal, so don't blame or chastise yourself. The main thing is to get back on track as swiftly as possible. This book offers science-based guidelines and lots of advice, but the important thing is that you fine-tune that advice so it works for you. Joining an online community of like-minded souls can be very helpful for keeping abreast of new science or simply sharing experiences.

Chapter eight

GETTING ACTIVE

Exercise is hugely important for health, particularly if you have difficulty controlling your blood sugar levels. As we have seen, the starting point for most type 2 diabetes is insulin resistance, where your body stops responding to insulin, forcing your pancreas to produce ever larger amounts of it. And the quickest and most effective way to reduce insulin resistance is to do more exercise.[47]

The problem is that many people find doing exercise a bit of a chore. This is a programme that will give you the maximum benefit in the minimum time.

The simplest of simple starts

The first and easiest thing you can do is stand every 30 minutes. You should start doing this from Week 1 of the diet. You might put this book down and do it right now.

The evidence that sitting kills goes back to the 1950s when a study was done comparing bus conductors (who stand) with bus drivers (who sit). It turned out that the bus drivers had twice the risk of developing heart disease.[48]

Since then we have become a lot more sedentary. We sit at work, in the car and at home, moving only to shift from one seat to another. Many of us spend more than half our waking lives, at least eight hours a day, sitting on our bottoms looking at computers or watching television.

The effects of this on our bodies are dire. One of the largest studies ever carried out,[49] involving nearly 800,000 people, found that those who are sedentary have:

- Twice the likelihood of developing type 2 diabetes

- Twice the likelihood of dying from a heart attack or stroke

Another way of putting this is that every hour you spend sitting down doing something like watching television cuts about 20 minutes off your life.[50]

It's not just the time spent sitting that matters but time spent sitting continuously. In a recent study from Australia,[51] researchers gathered 70 healthy adults and asked them to sit for nine hours. Every few hours they had to eat, and their blood sugar and insulin levels were measured. Then they did it all over again, except this time they got up every 30 minutes and walked around for a bit.

Just by standing up and walking every 30 minutes

they reduced their blood sugar levels by 39% and their insulin levels by 26%.

So get an app with an alarm that will remind you to move – every 30 minutes.

If you watch a lot of TV, set a timer and go for a stroll during the advert breaks. You could set an alarm that goes off in another room. Or keep the control beside the TV, so you have to get up to change channel. Television is designed to hook you in (I should know, I work in it) and the only way to combat its insidious charms is to be aware of its dangers.

Take a stand

If you are sitting less you are likely to be standing more. Many famous thinkers like Leonardo da Vinci and Ernest Hemingway found that they did their best work while standing.

But is it practical and how much difference would it make if we stood more? To find out I watched Dr John Buckley and a team of researchers from the University of Chester as they conducted a simple experiment.[52] They asked 10 people who work in an office to try standing for at least three hours a day for one week. Their normal desks were put away and replaced by special standing desks.

All the volunteers were equipped with accelerometers – movement monitors – to record just how much moving about they were doing. They also wore glucose monitors that measured their blood sugar levels constantly, day and night.

Some of the volunteers were nervous beforehand, saying things like "I think my feet might hurt", "My back won't stand it" or "I've never stood for as long as three hours."

In fact, they all stuck with it and one woman with arthritis found that standing actually improved her symptoms.

But what effects did it have on their bodies? Well, the first thing we discovered is the volunteers had much better control of their blood sugar. After eating a meal their blood sugar levels fell back to normal far more quickly than before.

They also burnt an extra 50 calories an hour. If you stand for three hours a day, for five days, that's around 750 calories a week. Over the course of a year it would add up to 30,000 extra calories, or around 8lb (3.5kg) of fat.

"That's the equivalent of running about 10 marathons a year," Dr Buckley says, "just by standing up three or four hours in your day."

We can't all stand up at work but even small adjustments, like standing while talking on the phone, going over to talk to a colleague rather than sending an email, will help.

Walk the walk

Even better than standing is walking. Walking is the great elixir of life and you should aim to do 10,000 steps a day. This is the minimum that is recommended to keep you healthy and help keep weight off.

In chapter six, in the "Before you start" section, I asked you to record how many steps you do over a typical week, so that you could monitor any increase.

You won't want to go from zero to 100mph, so aim for a steady build-up. Most people average around 5000 steps a day (those who are older and overweight tend to do less). If you increase the number of steps you do a day by 500 for every week you are on the BSD you should be close to the magic 10,000 by the end of eight weeks.

In other words, if you normally do 5000 steps a day, at the start of Week 1 you should aim to do 5500 steps a day, then in Week 2, 6000. And so on. You will find that as you lose weight you will become more energised and feel more willing to be active.

As you are going to be walking more you should invest in comfortable shoes. You may even want to buy special-ised walking socks with extra padding.

So how are you going to boost the number of steps you take? Ideally you will do it by building it into your day, so it is not a chore, just something you do without thinking.

My personal rules are:

1. I always take the stairs. I work on the seventh floor of a building in central London. It is 200 steps up and down. I do that at least twice a day. That comes to 800 steps.
2. I always walk or run on escalators.
3. When I am travelling around central London I always walk, if the journey is less than a mile, or I cycle if it is longer. I have a fold-up bike that I have spray-painted bright green so it is less likely to get stolen and I take it with me to work most days.
4. I live a mile from our local railway station, up a steep hill. I always cycle or walk to and from the station. Walking a mile is about 2000 steps.

Here are some other ways to build more steps into your life:

- Take public transport and get off the bus one stop earlier
- Listen to pacy music or an audio book – it can make walking more pleasurable.
- Leave your car at the far end of the car park when you go to the shops or supermarket.
- When you are at an airport, walk around rather than just sitting there, killing time. Walking before a flight helps with jetlag.

- When you are at work, pace around between meetings. Go and see colleagues rather than send emails. Stand while you are on the phone (research suggests this will also make you sound more assertive than when you are sitting).

- You might consider buying a treadmill desk. It allows you to walk while standing at your desk. It is not something I have ever attempted, but here's a link to a report by a BBC journalist who did give it a go: http://www.bbc.co.uk/news/magazine-21076461.

- Take up activities like gardening, painting or dancing, which require more movement.

- When you are on holiday, join a guided walking tour. They are normally in a group, last one to two hours, are very cheap, sometimes free, and led by knowledgeable, enthusiastic graduates. I've so far done this in Dublin, Berlin, London, Sydney and Paris. My kids, who really don't enjoy walking, are now very enthusiastic.

- Join a walking group or form your own. I have friends from Australia, Tim and Clare, and every year we aim to spend three or four days doing part of a classic English walk with them, such as the Coast to Coast (you walk from one side of England to the other). We do 10–12 miles a day and make a long weekend of it.

Tip: if you want to get maximum bang for your buck, then it is better to throw in a bit of fast walking rather than simply going for a gentle amble.

In a Danish study,[53] 32 diabetics were asked either to walk at a moderate pace for five hours a week, or to alternate three minutes' walking fast with three minutes' walking slow, again for five hours a week. After four months the group doing the fast-slow regime had lost an average of 6.6lb (3kg).

Strength training

Up until you're 30 your muscles get bigger. Then if you don't use them, they get smaller. You can lose 5% of your muscle mass every decade from age 30 onwards.

To keep your muscles you have to do some form of resistance training. You could go to the gym or do what I do, which is a simple regime designed to be done any time, any place.

With my regime you exercise as many major muscle

groups as possible, varying which ones each time, so the ones not being worked get a bit of a rest. I start with push-ups (working the upper body), and follow these with something that works the core (abdominal crunches) or the legs (squats).

What I do is based on a paper in the *American College of Sports Medicine's Health & Fitness Journal* [54] and I do it at least three times a week, first thing in the morning. It only takes a few minutes.

My favourite exercises are push-ups, squats, abdominal crunches, the bicep curl and the plank.

Push-ups: lie face down with the palms of your hands under your shoulders and the balls of your feet touching the ground. Keep your body straight. Lower your body till your elbows form a 90-degree angle and then push up. If you find this too hard, do it with your knees on the ground.

Squats: stand with your feet apart. Bend from the hips, keeping the weight in your heels. Make sure your back is straight. Keep bending until your legs are at a 90-degree angle – imagine you are preparing to sit in a chair. Push back up without bending your back. Squats work the biggest muscles in your body. If you are keen you can make this harder with weights.

Crunches: lie on your back with your knees bent, feet flat on the floor and your hands by the sides of your head. Curl up your upper body without lifting your lower back off the floor. Make sure your chin is tucked in towards your chest. When your shoulders and upper back are lifted off the floor, curl back down.

Bicep curls: this exercise requires small hand-held weights. You stand with your feet apart and your hands by your sides, with one hand clutching the small weight. Then, with your arm kept by your side, raise your hand by bending your elbow. Transfer the weight to your other hand and repeat.

Plank: lie face-down on the floor and then raise yourself on to your forearms and toes so that your body forms a straight line from head to toe. Make sure your mid-section doesn't rise or drop. Squeeze your buttocks and hold the position for as long as possible. Remember, it should never cause pain in the lower back.

I suggest you start by doing one set of 10 repeats of each of these in Week 1 of the diet (with 20-second holds on the planks). In other words: 10 press-ups, 10 crunches, 10 squats. Do this three times in the first week. Aim for two sets of 10 repeats by Week 2, and three sets by Week 4.

Getting more vigorous

The standard recommendations are to do at least 150 minutes of moderate aerobic activity (walking, swimming, mowing the lawn) or 75 minutes of vigorous aerobic activity (running, cycling, dancing) a week. Most of us don't get close.

That's why I like HIT (High Intensity Training), a completely different approach. It is short but intense. I do it at home but it is best, at least to start with, to do it in a supervised setting such as a gym. As with any other form of exercise, it would be wise to discuss with your doctor before starting, particularly if you are on medication.

High Intensity Training (HIT)

I was introduced to this form of exercise four years ago by Professor Jamie Timmons of Kings College, London. When I first met him he shocked me by saying that I could get most of the more important benefits of exercise from doing just three minutes a week of intensive cycling. I thought this sounded too good to be true, but I'm always up for a challenge, so I decided to give it a go.

Before I started they took some bloods and measured my fasting insulin and glucose. Then three times a week for the next six weeks I got on my exercise bike and pedalled away, following a regime that Professor Timmons recommended (see box on page 179). It was quite tough to start with, but I soon got used to it. My family also got used to the strange grunting noises I made as I pushed myself as hard as I could.

At the end of six weeks I went back to Prof Timmons' lab, had my bloods taken again and discovered that my insulin sensitivity had improved by an impressive 24%, which is broadly in line with what they expected (for some it will improve more, for others less).

So how does it work?

According to Jamie, if you are doing something very active, like HIT, you are breaking down the body's stores of glucose, deposited in your muscles as glycogen. Smash up these glycogen stores and you create room for more sugar to be sucked out of your blood after a meal.

Compared with standard exercise regimes, people who do HIT see a bigger loss in abdominal fat, which, as we've seen, is important because abdominal fat is so closely related to the risk of developing diabetes and heart disease.

A slow-build regime, for beginners
I like doing the 3 × 20-second regime, but unless you are already quite fit you should start with something that is less demanding. The following one is suggested for type 2 diabetics and those who are not particularly fit:

Week 1. You pedal away on an exercise bike for a few minutes. When you feel ready, you crank up the speed and pedal hard against resistance for 10 seconds. Then catch your breath and go back to pedalling slowly until 10 minutes are up. You do this three times in Week 1.

Week 2. You do the same, but this time you fit two "10-second bursts" into your 10-minute cycle ride. Each burst should be separated by a couple of minutes of gentle cycling, giving you time to recover.

Weeks 3 and 4. By now you should be able to push your short bursts up to 15 seconds. So you will be doing 2×15 seconds, within a 10-minute cycle ride, three times a week

Weeks 5 and 6. Try to do two lots of 20-second bursts in your 10-minute ride. You may be tempted to go on for longer than 20 seconds. Don't. Going for longer won't make it better and may make it worse.

Week 7 onwards. You can stick to two lots of 20 seconds. Or you can try moving on to three lots of 20 seconds. Just be sure that you are not pushing yourself too hard.

Michael's HIT regime

My regime consists of three bursts of 20 seconds, done three times a week on an exercise bike. You should only attempt this once you have built up some fitness. If you are unfit you should start by doing the beginner's regime I describe above.

1. Get on an exercise bike and do a short warm-up of gentle cycling, against limited resistance. You should just about notice the effort in your thighs.

2. After a couple of minutes, begin pedalling fast, then swiftly crank up the resistance.

The amount of resistance you select will depend on your strength and fitness. It should be high enough for you to feel it after 15 seconds of sprinting.

If, after 15 seconds, you can still keep going at the same pace without too much effort the resistance you've chosen isn't high enough. It mustn't, however, be so high that you grind to a complete halt. It's a matter of experimenting. What you'll find is that as you get fitter, the amount of resistance you can cope with increases. It's not speed but effort you are after.

3. After your first burst of fast sprinting, drop the resistance and do a couple of minutes of gentle pedalling to get your breath back.

4. Then do it twice more.

5. Finish with a couple of minutes of gentle cycling to allow your heart rate and blood pressure to return to normal before stepping off the bike.

In total this takes me less than 10 minutes.

Summary:

- Stand up every 30 minutes.

- Starting from your current level, add an extra 500 steps a day, each week, till you reach 10,000 steps a day.

- Do strength exercises three times a week, beginning slowly and adding in more reps each week.

- If you want to try HIT, it's best to start in a gym where you will be properly supervised.

Chapter nine

SORTING OUT YOUR HEAD

Stress and blood sugar problems are very strongly linked. High levels of the stress hormone, cortisol, make your muscles and other tissues more insulin-resistant. Stress reduces insulin's ability to get sugar into cells. Stress hormones also stimulate your liver to release more sugar into your blood.

Stress is an important cause of insomnia and weight gain too. When you feel stressed you are far more likely to give into carb cravings and comfort eating.

To keep weight off permanently you need to change the way you think about food and deal with setbacks. Many people who get their blood sugar back under control are changed by the experience. Remember Carlos? He was so sick he thought he was about to die. Now he works with overeaters as a diabetes buddy. Geoff Whitington is also a diabetes champion – audiences love him because they can relate to his experiences. Bob Smietana, the Chicago journalist who regularly ate doughnuts for breakfast, is training to run marathons. They have sustained their weight loss by making it part of who they are and reminding themselves how far they have come.

Cassie, the trainee nurse, put it powerfully when she wrote, "It is the best feeling in the world not having to take insulin any more. Every time I'm tempted to eat something I shouldn't I say to myself, 'If you eat that then you will be back on insulin' and the temptation goes. I have been in a food prison for so long: thinking about what I want to eat and then, when I've eaten it, feeling guilty about what I've just eaten. I don't do that any more. I now think about life and living and I get so much more done!"

That said, there are always going to be difficult and stressful days when things are going badly and you reach for a large tub of ice cream or a family-sized bar of chocolate. If you give in (and most of us will at some point in our lives), then beware of a common dieting pitfall, "catastrophic thinking".

Imagine, for whatever reasons, you have a bit of a splurge. Instead of thinking, "That was a one-off, I'm only human", you say to yourself, "I'm a weak-willed failure, I will never succeed, I'm never going to be able to stay off sugar. I might as well give up now." The results of giving into catastrophic thinking can be catastrophic gorging.

I recently saw a TV experiment in which a group of dieters were divided into two teams and then, separately, taken along to a cake-making lesson.

Just before they started, Team A were offered a slice of

cake. After they had eaten it they were told they had just eaten 750 calories.

Team B were offered a slice of the same cake, but they were told that the slice they had eaten was only 190 calories.

Then both teams spent an afternoon making cakes while being secretly filmed.

Team A, who felt they had already blown their diet, decided "what the hell", and began eating any spare cakes they could hoover up. They ended up eating almost 4.4lb (2kg) of cake between just four of them. Team B, who thought they'd only had a modest treat, were much more restrained, and though they ate some extra cake, it was far less.

The lesson is: watch out for tricky psychologists. But also watch out for catastrophic thinking, One way to counter it is to be aware you are doing it. Another way is to practise mindfulness.

Mindfulness – reducing stress

Many of us go through life with self-critical and unhelpful thoughts rattling around inside our heads, each thought competing for our attention. These constant mental meanderings can lead to a spiral of over-eating, self-loathing, depression and insomnia.

Saying, "Pull yourself together" rarely works. But you

can counter these negative thoughts by making yourself more "mindful". Instead of obsessing, take time out to look at yourself and your thoughts in a less judgmental, more reasonable way.

Mindfulness is a modern take on the ancient practice of meditation. The good news is you don't need to be religious or go on a retreat to a Tibetan monastery to do it.

You can buy books about mindfulness, but it's not really something you need to read about; it's something you need to do. I recommend joining a group or downloading an app like "Headspace", which was created by a former monk, Andy Puddicombe, and will guide you through the process.

The app sessions are short – at first it's just 10 minutes, then 15 minutes, and finally 20 minutes, so it's not a particularly time-consuming thing to do. You may be cynical, but it really is worth trying. I find it reduces cravings and helps me sleep better.

When I'm doing a mindfulness session I sit in a comfortable chair, turn on my app, rest my hands on my thighs and close my eyes. Then, guided by the app, I spend the next few minutes trying to focus of my breath.

I pay attention to the sensation of the breath going through my nostrils, filling my chest, expanding and contracting my diaphragm. I try to stay focused on this task and when I notice that my thoughts have drifted, which they do, I bring them back to my breath.

I try to treat thoughts like balloons that drift into my

consciousness; once I have noticed they are there I simply allow them to drift way.

I say "simply", but when you first start you will find it's almost impossible to stop thinking about deadlines, food, the overdraft, the kids, your ex-partner, etc... You might start thinking, "This isn't working, what is Michael Mosley on about?" Put those suspicious thoughts aside; it will get easier. Like any skill, practice makes perfect.

Mindfulness can be very effective in a surprisingly short time. In a recent study,[55] researchers took 15 volunteers who had never tried anything like mindfulness and put them through a brain scanner. They also got them to fill in an anxiety questionnaire.

The volunteers then did four sessions of mindfulness training, spread over four days, and the tests were repeated. Anxiety ratings fell by 39%. The results also showed that activity also increased in the areas of the brain that control worrying, particularly the ventromedial prefrontal cortex and the anterior cingulate gyrus. This supports the claim that mindfulness strengthens our ability to ignore negative thoughts and feelings.

To get a flavour of what mindfulness can do you could try either or both of the following:

Breathing exercise
Go into a quiet room and sit with your eyes closed. Breathe in and out of your nose, slowly counting to four as you inhale and again to four as you exhale. Use very

shallow breathes; don't let your chest rise and fall. Set a timer and do this for three minutes.

Progressive muscle relaxation
In the 1920s, Dr Edmund Jacobson developed a technique of tensing and totally relaxing specific muscle groups. A study published in *Diabetes Care* showed that five weekly sessions of this kind of therapy helped to reduce blood sugar levels. It is easiest if someone guides you through it, rather than trying to do it and read this book at the same time! Or you can just record your own voice instructing you what to do.

> *Sit in a chair with your feet flat on the floor. Close your eyes. When you tense a muscle, hold the tension for five seconds and then relax for 30 seconds before you go on to the next tensing movement. After you are done, breathe in deeply and stretch.*
>
> *Right hand and forearm:* make a fist and then release.
>
> *Right upper arm:* bend your arm to tense the muscle, then release.
>
> *Left hand and forearm:* make a fist and then release.
>
> *Left upper arm:* bend your arm to tense the muscle, then release.

Forehead: raise your eyebrows and then relax your face.

Eye and cheeks: squeeze your eyes shut and then relax.

Mouth and jaw: clench your teeth and pull the corners of your mouth down and relax.

Shoulder and neck: lock your hands behind your neck and push the back of your head against this resistance (don't move your head). Pull up your shoulders and press your head back against their resistance in a horizontal movement.

Chest and back: breathe in deeply and hold your breath, pressing your shoulders together at the back at the same time, then let your shoulders hang, and breathe normally.

Belly: tighten your abs and then release

Right thigh: move your right foot forward against resistance and then release.

Right calf: lift up your right heel and then relax.

Right foot: bend your toes and then release.

Left thigh: move your left foot forward and relax.

Left calf: lift up your left heel and then relax.

Left foot: bend your toes and then relax.

GOING FORWARD

So that's it – quite a lot to digest. Rising blood sugar is a serious threat but I am greatly encouraged by the work that is being done showing how we can combat and reverse it.

The link with fat is clear; not so much the fat in our diet as the fat in our midriffs, tummy fat, visceral fat, the fat that infiltrates your liver and your pancreas. Get rid of that (or preferably stop it building up in the first place) and so many problems get sorted.

There are lots of reasons why we are where we are, including the way that the food industry responded to the low-fat diet message by pumping products full of sugar instead. There is evidence that the tide is turning, with consumers saying that added sugars are one of their biggest concerns.

But I also think that we, collectively as a society I think, have to change the mindset that says that it's OK to give ourselves, and our children, endless little treats. Snacking is not just a guilty pleasure – it's helping drive the diabesity epidemic.

If you've got type 2 diabetes, prediabetes or just high

blood sugar, then the message of this book is clear: *do something about it*. Don't assume that drugs will make it better or that your doctor has all the answers. If you've been wondering whether you might have blood sugar problems or if you have a friend or relative you think might be at risk, do get tested. The longer you leave it, the worse things get.

Pharmaceutical companies are beavering away developing new drugs. Surgeons are perfecting and promoting operations for weight loss. That is where a lot of research money is going.

But I believe that many people, given the choice, would rather heal themselves, through weight loss and diet. One of the things that has thrilled me most over the two years that I've been working on this book has been the inspiring stories of change, from people who have turned their lives around.

This book contains everything you need to know to do the 8-week Blood Sugar Diet. But if you would like more information, advice or support, please go to www. thebloodsugardiet.com

It's early days for this site and we would greatly appreciate feedback. We want to help build a community where people share experiences and recipes and support each other through the difficult times. It will include the latest research and up-to-date advice for professionals and dieters alike.

RECIPES AND MENU PLANS

by Dr Sarah Schenker

1. 50 recipes for breakfast, brunch, lunch & supper
2. Quick and easy recipes
3. Instant soups
4. Guilt-free baking
5. Menu plans

NB. For the sake of simplicity, all calorie counts have been rounded up or down to the nearest 10.

All calorie counts are for one portion

50 RECIPES FOR BREAKFAST, BRUNCH, LUNCH & SUPPER

Breakfast
(less than 200 calories)

Yoghurt 3 ways

Rhubarb compote – 160 calories
Serves 1

500g rhubarb, trimmed and cut into small chunks
Zest and juice of 1 orange
Zest and juice of 1 lemon
Knob of root ginger, peeled and finely chopped
150g plain yoghurt

Preheat the oven to 180°C/gas mark 4. Put the rhubarb, orange and lemon zest and juice and ginger in an oven-proof dish. Cook in the oven, uncovered, for 30–40 minutes. Allow to cool and then transfer to an airtight container. This will keep in the fridge for 1–2 days.

Swirl 2 tbsp of the rhubarb through the yoghurt.

Passion fruit and almonds – 170 calories
Serves 1

150g plain yoghurt
1 tbsp flaked almonds
1 passion fruit

Toast the flaked almonds in a dry frying pan over a low heat for a few minutes, until they turn golden. Remove from the pan and allow to cool.

Tip the yoghurt into a bowl and stir in the almonds. Cut the passion fruit in half, scoop out the seeds and stir them into the yoghurt.

Apple, mango and hazelnut – 180 calories
Serves 1

150g plain yoghurt
1 apple, cored and diced
½ mango, peeled and cut into chunks
1 tbsp skinned hazelnuts

Place the mango and hazelnuts in a food processor and pulse a few times to form a rough paste. Place in the bottom of a dish, add the chunks of apple and top with the yoghurt.

Almond butter with apple, seeds and goji berries – 110 calories

Makes 4 portions of almond butter

For the butter:
100g skin-on almonds

2 tsp mixed seeds and goji berries
1 apple, cored and sliced

To make the almond butter, preheat the oven to 190°C/ gas mark 5 and place the almonds on a baking sheet and bake in the oven for 10 minutes. Remove from the oven and allow to cool. Then place in a food processor and blitz until smooth. (The butter keeps in the fridge for 2–3 days.)

Serve 2 tbsp of the butter in a dish and sprinkle with the mixed seeds and goji berries; add apple wedges for dipping.

Portobello 'toast' with wilted spinach and chickpeas – 150 calories

Serves 1

2 portobello mushrooms
Drizzle of olive oil
2 handfuls of spinach
2 tbsp tinned chickpeas, drained and rinsed
Pinch of nutmeg
Pinch of paprika

Turn the grill to high. Place the mushrooms on the baking tray, drizzle with the oil and season with a pinch of salt and plenty of black pepper. Place under the grill for 3 minutes.

Meanwhile place the spinach in a small pan with a splash of water and cook it on a medium heat until it has wilted. Drain and sprinkle with the nutmeg.

Place the chickpeas in a bowl, sprinkle with the paprika and roughly mash with a fork. Divide the spinach and chickpeas between the 2 mushrooms.

Portobello 'toast' with goat's cheese and pine nuts – 150 calories
Serves 1

2 portobello mushrooms
Drizzle of olive oil
30g goat's cheese
1 tbsp pine nuts
Handful of chives, snipped

Turn the grill to high. Place the mushrooms on the baking tray, drizzle with the oil and season with a pinch of salt and plenty of black pepper. Place under the grill for 3 minutes. Remove the mushrooms from the grill, dot on the cheese and sprinkle on the pine nuts. Return the mushrooms to the grill for a further 2 minutes. Sprinkle on the chives.

No-carb bircher – 180 calories
Serves 1

1 tbsp raisins
50ml apple juice
2 tbsp ground flaxseed
2 tbsp plain yoghurt
Pinch of ground cinnamon
1 tbsp walnut pieces

Place the raisins in a bowl and pour over the apple juice. Leave to chill in the fridge for at least 1 hour or overnight.

When ready to eat, mix with the ground flaxseed and the yoghurt and sprinkle over the cinnamon and walnut pieces.

Spinach and pea omelette – 180 calories
Serves 1

50g frozen peas
Large handful of spinach
2 eggs
1 tbsp chives, snipped
Drizzle of olive oil

Bring a pan of water to the boil and cook the peas for 5 minutes. Add the spinach for the last minute and then drain well.

Whisk the eggs together and season well. Add the peas, spinach and chives and mix well. Heat the oil in a pan, add the egg mixture and cook through.

Grilled apricots with yoghurt – 140 calories
Serves 2

For the marinade:
1 tsp olive oil
1 tbsp fresh lime juice
1 tsp ground cinnamon

6 apricots, peeled and cut into 1cm slices
4 tbsp Greek yoghurt
50g raspberries
1 tbsp hazelnuts, roughly chopped
Handful of mint leaves, torn

In a small bowl, combine the olive oil, lime juice and cinnamon and whisk to blend. Set aside.

Lightly brush the apricots with the marinade. Place under a hot grill, turning once and basting once or twice with the remaining marinade, until tender and golden, about 3–5 minutes on each side.

Serve with the yoghurt, scattered with the raspberries, hazelnuts and mint.

Melon, spinach and blueberry shake – 130 calories
Serves 1

¼ Galia melon, chopped
50g blueberries
200ml unsweetened almond milk
2 handfuls of baby spinach leaves
Sprinkle of sunflower seeds

Put the melon, berries, spinach and almond milk into a blender and whizz until smooth. Stir in the sunflower seeds and pour into a container or flask. Leave to chill in the fridge for at least an hour (this is fine to make the night before).

Blueberry and green tea shake – 100 calories
Serves 1

200ml water
1 green teabag
50g blueberries
2 tbsp Greek yoghurt
1 tbsp almonds
1 tbsp flaxseeds

Bring the water to the boil and add the teabag and allow it to steep for 4 minutes. Remove the teabag and chill the tea in the fridge (preferably overnight). Pour into a blender with the other ingredients and whizz together.

2 × green "drinks"
Serves 1

Spinach and raspberry – 70 calories

2 large handfuls of baby spinach leaves
200ml coconut water
Handful of raspberries
Juice of 1 lime

Blend everything together and serve chilled.

3 cup mix – approx 90 calories

1 cup of green veg (e.g. chard, pak choi, spinach,
  kale, courgette)
1 cup of liquid: either coconut water, almond milk,
  or plain yoghurt diluted with water to taste
1 cup of fruit: apple, berries or orange

Blend the leafy veg and the liquid together; then add the
fruit and blend again.

This can be frozen, or stored in the fridge for 1 day.

Brunch

(higher calorie count: 300–400 calories)

Veg frittata – 320 calories
Serves 2

2 red peppers
Drizzle of olive oil
3 spring onions, chopped
2 garlic cloves, crushed
½ × 400g tin chickpeas, drained and rinsed
1 tsp smoked paprika
100g baby spinach leaves
4 large eggs, beaten
Pinch of salt and freshly ground black pepper

Cut the peppers and into halves or quarters and remove the seeds. Brush lightly with oil, then place the pieces skin side up on a baking sheet and grill on high, until the skin blackens and blisters. Place the hot peppers in a heatproof bag and seal tightly. Leave to cool. Peel the charred skin from the peppers and roughly chop.

Heat the olive oil in a large frying pan over a medium heat and sauté the spring onions and garlic until soft. Add the pepper to the pan, with the chickpeas and paprika. Sauté everything together for about 5 minutes.

Add the spinach and keep stirring until it wilts. Add

the eggs and seasoning and stir gently to incorporate them into the whole mixture, then allow to set over a medium heat – this should take just 2 minutes.

Preheat the grill to high, then slide the whole pan underneath to set the top of the frittata. It will only take a minute to become light golden and puffed up.

No-carb waffles – 290 calories
Makes 2 waffles = 1 serving

2 egg whites plus 1 whole egg
2 tbsp coconut flour
2 tbsp milk
½ tsp baking powder
Oil spray
A few strawberries to serve

Whip the egg whites to stiff peaks. Stir in the coconut flour, milk, baking powder and the whole egg.

Heat up your waffle iron to the highest temperature, and grease or spray it with non-stick spray. Pour in the batter, and cook until browned, about 3–4 minutes. (If you don't have a waffle iron, a hot frying pan will do; spray the pan with oil, and then use a ladle to pour half of the mixture to make a thick pancake.) Serve with the strawberries.

Baked eggs with minted pea and feta salad – 330 calories
Serves 4

Butter for greasing
3 large eggs
125ml half-fat crème fraîche
1 tbsp grated Parmesan cheese
Handful of fresh basil leaves, torn
300g peas
3 tbsp fresh mint, chopped
1 avocado, diced
Juice of 1 lemon
1 tbsp olive oil
50g spinach leaves
100g feta, crumbled

Preheat the oven to 180°C/gas mark 4 and grease 4 holes of a 12-hole muffin tray with the butter.

Whisk the eggs, crème fraîche, Parmesan and basil leaves together in a bowl until well combined and season to taste with salt and freshly ground black pepper. Divide the mixture between the muffin holes and bake in the oven for 10–12 minutes, until the eggs are just set.

Meanwhile, mix the peas, mint, avocado, lemon juice and olive oil in a bowl.

To serve, divide the spinach between 4 plates and spoon some pea and mint salad on top. Sprinkle over the crumbled feta and serve with the baked eggs.

Mexican hash – 340 calories
Serves 2

1 red chilli, slit lengthways and deseeded
1 tbsp rapeseed oil
200g baby mushrooms, halved
1 garlic clove, chopped
1 tsp Cajun seasoning
200g tin black beans, drained and rinsed
2 eggs
1 ripe avocado, chopped
Lime wedges
Salt and freshly ground black pepper

Slice half the chilli into strips and set aside; finely chop the other half.

Heat the rapeseed oil in a pan over a medium heat and fry the mushrooms for about 5 minutes or until golden. Add the chopped chilli, garlic, Cajun seasoning and black beans and heat through for about 5 minutes; season to taste. Keep warm while you fry the eggs.

Use the same frying pan with the residual oil to fry the eggs until cooked to your liking.

Divide the mushroom mixture between 2 bowls and top each one with a fried egg, some chopped avocado and the sliced chilli. Serve with the lime wedges.

Skinny kedgeree – 360 calories
Serves 2

1 large cauliflower
1 tbsp olive oil
1 small red onion, chopped
1 red chilli, deseeded and chopped
2 tbsp medium curry powder
1 tsp mustard seeds
1 tsp cayenne pepper
2 small smoked mackerel fillets, flaked
2 eggs, hardboiled
4 spring onions, sliced
Handful of flat-leaf parsley, chopped
Salt and freshly ground black pepper

To make the cauliflower "rice": preheat the oven to 200°C/ gas mark 6. Discard the stalk and place the florets in a food processor and blitz for 30 seconds. Transfer to a bowl and then add a drizzle of olive oil and toss gently. Spread the blitzed cauliflower out in a thin layer on a baking tray and bake for 10 minutes.

Meanwhile, put the rest of the oil in a non-stick frying pan over a medium heat and soften the onion and chilli for 5 minutes. Add all the spices and fry for a further 1–2 minutes.

Stir the cauliflower into the onion mixture and then add the mackerel. Season well and heat through gently for a few minutes.

Peel and quarter the boiled eggs. Stir the spring onions

and parsley into the cauliflower mixture, divide between 2 bowls and top with the egg quarters.

Poached egg and salmon stack – 320 calories
Serves 2

4 portobello mushrooms
Drizzle of olive oil
2 slices (approx 50g) of smoked salmon
1 tbsp half-fat crème fraîche
1 tsp wholegrain mustard
Squeeze of lemon juice
2 handfuls of watercress, chopped
2 eggs, poached
1 tbsp pine nuts, toasted

Turn the grill to high. Place the mushrooms on the baking tray, drizzle with the oil and season with a pinch of salt and plenty of black pepper. Grill for 3 minutes.

Put a slice of smoked salmon on each mushroom. Mix together the crème fraîche, mustard and lemon juice and spread over the salmon.

Top with a handful of watercress, a poached egg and a scattering of pine nuts.

Soups, salads and lunches
(200–300 calories)

Lettuce cups 3 ways
Serves 1

Separate the leaves of a gem lettuce and add a dollop of any of the following fillings to each leaf.

Crab and mustard – 210 calories
Mix 100g white crab meat with 1 tbsp crème fraîche, 1 tsp Dijon mustard, a squeeze of lemon juice, a small handful of chopped dill and 1 tsp capers.

Chicken and walnut – 300 calories
Mix 1 tbsp crème fraîche with 1 tsp Dijon mustard and a squeeze of lemon juice. Add 100g cooked chicken pieces, along with a small red apple (cored and sliced), 1 tbsp walnut pieces and a chopped celery stick.

Bacon and avocado – 290 calories
Grill 2 rashers of lean back bacon, and when cool enough to handle cut into fine strips. Add the flesh of half an avocado and a diced radish. Use the back of a spoon to combine together gently so the bacon and radish are held in the crushed avocado.

Chicken, butterbean and walnut salad – 270 calories
Serves 2

200g chicken breast, diced
2 sprigs of rosemary, leaves picked and finely chopped
1 garlic clove, finely chopped
Drizzle of olive oil
50g green beans, trimmed
100g tinned butter beans, drained and rinsed
1 red onion, very thinly sliced
1 tbsp walnut pieces

For the dressing:
1 tbsp olive oil
1 tbsp wholegrain mustard
1 tbsp white wine vinegar

Place the chicken, rosemary and garlic in a large bowl, drizzle with a little olive oil and toss together. Put a large non-stick frying pan on a medium-high heat and add the chicken pieces. Cook, stirring, for about 10 minutes or until the chicken is browned and cooked through. Meanwhile, bring a large pan of water to the boil and add the green beans. Boil for 2 minutes, then add the butter beans and cook for a further 2 minutes. The green beans should be tender and the butter beans heated through. Drain well.

In a large serving bowl, mix together the warm chicken, beans, red onion and walnuts. To make the dressing, whisk together the oil, mustard and vinegar in a small bowl. Pour over the salad and toss gently to combine.

Crayfish salad – 250 calories

Serves 1

For the dressing (enough for 2–3 portions):
1 small shallot
1 garlic clove
½ red chilli
1 tbsp olive oil
1 tbsp fish sauce
Juice of 1 lemon
1 tbsp white wine vinegar

100g crayfish
4 radishes, halved
¼ cucumber, diced
1 celery stick, chopped
2 large handfuls of rocket

Make the dressing by finely chopping the shallot, garlic and chilli and placing in a jam jar with the oil, fish sauce, lemon juice and vinegar. Secure the lid and shake well to combine.

Arrange the crayfish in a bowl with the vegetables and dress with 1 tbsp of the dressing.

Courgette and feta salad – 270 calories

Serves 1

1 courgette
2 large handfuls of rocket
50g raspberries

1 tbsp olive oil
1 tbsp balsamic vinegar
40g feta, diced
1 tbsp pumpkin seeds
Handful of mint leaves, torn

Peel a courgette into long ribbons using a spiraliser or potato peeler. Mix with the rocket and raspberries. Drizzle with olive oil and balsamic vinegar and top with the feta, pumpkin seeds and some torn mint leaves.

Beetroot falafels – 290 calories
Serves 2

½ tbsp olive oil
1 red onion, chopped
1 tsp cumin seeds
Pinch of cayenne pepper
4 mushrooms, finely chopped
1 × 400g tin chickpeas, drained and rinsed
250g raw beetroot, peeled and coarsely grated
1 egg
1 tbsp tahini paste
Squeeze of lemon juice
Vegetable oil, for brushing

To serve:
2 tbsp Greek yoghurt
1 bag of rocket leaves

Preheat the oven to 200°C/gas mark 6.

Heat the oil in a frying pan and fry the onions for 5 minutes or until softened. Add the cumin, cayenne and mushrooms and cook for another 2 minutes, then transfer the mixture to a food processor with the chickpeas, two-thirds of the grated beetroot, egg, tahini and lemon juice. Whizz to a rough paste, transfer to a bowl and stir in the remaining grated beetroot. Season with a pinch of salt and plenty of black pepper.

With damp hands, shape the mixture into 8 balls and space on a baking sheet lined with parchment. Brush the falafels with a little oil and bake for 25 minutes.

Serve them with a dollop of Greek yoghurt and a handful of rocket.

Pepper with jewelled feta – 220 calories
Serves 1

1 red pepper
25g feta, diced
1 tbsp mint, roughly chopped
1 tbsp coriander, roughly chopped
1 spring onion, finely chopped
1 tbsp pistachio nuts, roughly chopped
4 cherry tomatoes, halved
5cm piece of cucumber, diced
Seeds from a pomegranate
Juice of half a lemon

Cut the pepper in half and remove the seeds. Brush the skin with some olive oil and place the pieces skin side up on a baking tray. Heat the grill to high and place the pepper under for 5 minutes.

Place all the other ingredients in a bowl or tub and toss together.

Remove the pepper halves from the grill and stuff with the feta mixture.

Beetroot, apple and cannellini bean soup – 200 calories
Makes 3 portions; can be kept in the fridge for 3 days or in the freezer for up to a month

1 tbsp olive oil
1 tsp cumin seeds
2 medium onions, roughly chopped
500g raw beetroot, grated
2 Bramley apples, peeled and quartered
1 litre chicken or vegetable stock
2 star anise
Salt and freshly ground black pepper
1 × 400g tin cannellini beans, drained and rinsed
Greek yoghurt, to serve
Handful of chives, chopped

Heat the oil in a large saucepan, then add the cumin seeds and onions, and cook gently for 10 minutes with the lid on. Add the grated beetroot and apple, stir well, replace the lid and cook for a further 10 minutes. Pour in the stock, turn the heat up, add the star anise and season with a pinch of salt and plenty of black pepper. Bring to the boil and simmer for 5 minutes.

Remove from the heat, take out the star anise and blitz the soup in a blender until puréed. Return to the pan, add the beans and allow to simmer for 20 minutes. Serve with a swirl of Greek yoghurt and some chopped chives.

Hummus 3 ways
Each recipe makes 3 portions and can be kept in the fridge for 2–3 days

Classic spicy – 250 calories

1 × 400g tin chickpeas, drained and rinsed
Juice of half a lemon
1 garlic clove
1 tsp paprika
2 tbsp olive oil
2 tbsp tahini paste

Whizz everything together in a blender until smooth. Loosen with a little water if the mixture is too thick.

Beetroot hummus – 200 calories

250g raw beetroot
2 × 400g tins chickpeas, drained and rinsed
Juice of 1 lemon

1 tsp ground cumin
Salt and pepper
2 tbsp Greek yoghurt

Cook the beetroot in a large pan of boiling water with the lid on for 30–40 mins, or until tender. When they're done, a skewer or knife should go all the way in easily. Drain, then set aside to cool.

When cool enough to handle, peel and roughly chop the flesh, then place in a food processor and whizz together with the chickpeas, lemon juice, cumin, a pinch of salt and some pepper. Transfer to a bowl and swirl through the yoghurt.

Minted pea hummus – 170 calories

200g cooked peas
1 garlic clove, crushed
1 tbsp tahini
Squeeze of lemon juice
1 tbsp tinned chickpeas
2 tbsp olive oil
Handful of mint leaves

Place all the ingredients in a food processor and blitz together to form a thick paste. Add 1–2 tbsp water, then blitz again.

Chickpea and hazelnut salad – 270 calories
Serves 2

100g butternut squash, peeled and diced
1 tbsp olive oil
½ tsp allspice
80g green beans
200g tinned chickpeas, drained and rinsed
1 tbsp hazelnuts
2 handfuls of watercress leaves
8 cherry tomatoes, halved
2 spring onions, chopped
½ cucumber, chopped
1 tbsp balsamic vinegar

Preheat the oven to 190°C/gas mark 5. Place the butternut squash in a pan, cover with boiling water and simmer for 5 minutes, then drain well and spread out on a baking sheet.

Drizzle with half the olive oil and sprinkle on the allspice. Bake in the oven until golden, about 15 minutes.

Steam the green beans and set aside.

Transfer the baked butternut squash to a bowl and add the chickpeas, hazelnuts, watercress, tomatoes, spring onions, cucumber and beans. Toss together and dress with the remaining olive oil and balsamic vinegar.

Spanish chickpea and spinach soup – 210 calories
Makes 2 portions

50g Spanish chorizo, diced
1 tbsp olive oil
1 large leek, thinly sliced
2 medium garlic cloves, finely chopped
1 red pepper, diced
Pinch of chilli flakes
1 tsp paprika
1 tbsp tomato purée
1 litre chicken stock
200g tinned chickpeas, drained and rinsed
150g baby spinach

Place a small non-stick pan over a medium heat and add the chorizo. Cook, stirring occasionally, for about 5 minutes, until most of the fat melts out. Set aside to drain on paper towels and discard the fat.

Add the olive oil to a large pan and place over a medium heat. Add the leek and cook, stirring frequently, for about 5 minutes, then the garlic, pepper, chilli flakes and paprika and cook for a further minute. Add the tomato purée and cook, stirring frequently, for 2 more minutes. Pour in the stock and chickpeas and bring to the boil.

Reduce the heat to a simmer, partially cover and cook for 20 minutes.

Finally, put in the baby spinach leaves and the cooked chorizo and heat through until the spinach is wilted.

Prawn pho – 170 calories
Makes 2 portions

1 litre vegetable stock
50g baby sweetcorn
Handful of bean sprouts
50g mange tout
50g sugar snap peas
Knob of ginger, peeled and grated
1 tbsp fish sauce
Juice of half a lime
12 large prawns, shelled and deveined
Handful each of fresh basil, mint, coriander
½ red chilli, finely sliced

Pour the stock into a large saucepan and bring to the boil.
Add the sweetcorn, bean sprouts, mange tout, peas and
ginger and cook for 3–4 minutes. Add the fish sauce and
lime juice, and season. Cook the prawns in the broth till
pink, about 2–3 minutes. Serve topped with the herbs
and red chilli.

Ricotta, pear and walnut salad – 290 calories
Serves 1

50g fresh ricotta
2 spring onions, finely chopped
50g green beans
1 tbsp olive oil
1 tbsp lemon juice

½ garlic clove, crushed
Handful of flat-leaf parsley, chopped
Pinch of nutmeg
2 large handfuls of watercress
1 small pear, quartered
1 tbsp walnut pieces

Crumble the ricotta into a bowl, add the spring onions and gently toss together.

Place the green beans in a small pan of boiling water, cook for 3–4 minutes. Drain well, refresh under cold running water and set aside.

To make the salad dressing, whisk the oil, lemon juice, garlic, parsley and nutmeg in a bowl, then season.

Arrange the watercress, green beans and pear in a dish, add the ricotta and spring onion mixture, drizzle over the dressing and scatter on the walnuts.

Skinny spicy bean burgers – 280 calories

Makes 4 burgers = 2 servings (the mixture can be kept chilled in the fridge for 2–3 days)

4 mushrooms
Handful of fresh coriander
1 × 400g tin of cannellini beans, drained and rinsed
1 × 400g tin of kidney beans, drained and rinsed
1 egg
½ onion, finely chopped
1 chilli, finely sliced

1 tsp ground coriander
1 tsp ground cumin
1 tsp paprika
1 tsp chilli powder or a few drops of Tabasco sauce
Drizzle of olive oil
Flour for dusting
Bag of mixed salad leaves
1 beef tomato to serve

Place the mushrooms and coriander in a food processor and blitz till they resemble breadcrumbs. Then add the beans and egg and blend together to form a chunky mixture.

Stir in the rest of the ingredients until combined. Dust your hands with flour and shape the mixture into 4 burgers.

Heat a drizzle of olive oil in a large pan and fry the burgers over a medium heat until brown and hot all the way through. Serve with handfuls of mixed leaves and thick slices of the tomato.

Chicken and asparagus salad – 270 calories
Serves 2

2 skinless chicken breasts
1 bundle of asparagus (about 200g), tough ends snapped
  off and discarded
1 red pepper, deseeded and thinly sliced
Olive oil, for drizzling

Salt and black pepper
2 tbsp plain yoghurt
1 tbsp sour cream
1 tbsp white wine vinegar
½ garlic clove, crushed
1 tbsp chopped dill
120g bag of mixed salad leaves
2 tbsp pine nuts, toasted

Preheat the oven to 220°C/gas mark 7. Arrange the chicken, asparagus and red pepper in a large, shallow roasting tin and drizzle with olive oil. Season well and then roast in the oven for 20 minutes, stirring halfway through, or until the chicken is cooked through and the vegetables are tender and starting to caramelise.

In a small bowl, whisk together the yoghurt, sour cream, vinegar, garlic and dill to make a dressing. Season to taste.

Divide the salad leaves between 2 plates, scatter over the pine nuts and arrange the chicken and vegetables on top. Serve with the dressing.

Warm halloumi salad – 280 calories
Serves 2

½ tsp chilli powder
Large handful of mint leaves, chopped
Zest and juice of half a lemon
1 tbsp olive oil

1 courgette, cut into 1cm rounds
150g pack halloumi cheese, cubed
4 handfuls of rocket leaves
1 red pepper, deseeded and diced
1 tbsp sliced black olives

Mix together the chilli, half the mint, lemon zest and juice, oil, courgette and halloumi. Leave to marinate for 30 minutes. Soak 8 wooden skewers in water for 20 minutes.

Thread the courgettes and halloumi onto the skewers, and put the remaining marinade to one side. Cook on the BBQ, or under a grill, for 7–8 minutes, turning halfway through and basting with a bit of the remaining marinade.

Place the rocket in a bowl with the pepper, olives and remaining mint and dress with the last of the marinade.

Grapefruit and Manchego salad – 280 calories
Serves 2

1 large pink grapefruit
80g Manchego cheese (or Cheddar), diced
1 avocado, diced
½ fennel bulb, thinly sliced
Juice of 1 lime
1 tbsp olive oil
1 tbsp balsamic vinegar
Large handful of fresh coriander, chopped

Peel the grapefruit and separate the segments with a knife, catching the juice in a bowl. Place the cheese, avocado and fennel, the grapefruit and its juice in the bowl and toss together. Make up the dressing by mixing the lime juice, oil and vinegar together. Pour over the salad and sprinkle on the fresh coriander.

Supper
(350–500 calories)

Luxury fish pie with celeriac topping – 470 calories
Serves 4

For the mash topping:
2 small celeriacs, peeled and diced
1 tbsp milk
1 tbsp butter
Salt and pepper

Drizzle of olive oil
1 large onion, finely diced
2 leeks, finely sliced
2 tbsp fresh parsley, chopped
1 tbsp fresh dill, chopped
100g mushrooms, chopped
400g sustainable white fish fillets (e.g.

haddock, cod, coley), cut into chunks
150g peeled prawns
1 bay leaf
250ml milk

Preheat the oven to 180°C/gas mark 4. Make the mash by boiling the celeriac until tender, about 10 minutes. Drain and transfer to a blender, add a little milk, a knob of butter and some salt and pepper and whizz to a purée. Put to one side in a bowl.

Heat the olive oil in a large pan and cook the onion, leeks and herbs for a few mins. Set aside on a plate. In the same frying pan, cook the mushrooms for a few minutes until lightly golden. Add them to the onion and leek mixture.

Place the fish and prawns in a large pan, add the milk and the bay leaf and bring to the boil. Poach for about 4 minutes, then lift out the fish and prawns with a slotted spoon. Keep the milk, removing any bones or skin and the bay leaf.

Arrange the fish on the bottom of an ovenproof serving dish and put the mushroom, onion and leek mixture on top. Pour over 3–4 tbsp of the cooking milk to add some moisture to the dish.

Cover with the mashed celeriac. Cook in the oven for 15 minutes.

Courgetti prawns – 390 calories
Serves 2

1 leek (or 2 baby leeks), thickly sliced
1 courgette, spiralised or cut into ribbons with a peeler
2cm piece of root ginger, peeled and grated
½ red chilli, chopped
1 garlic clove, crushed
Juice of 1 lemon
1 tbsp olive oil
200g raw prawns
½ × 400g tin cannellini beans, drained and rinsed
2 handfuls of fresh coriander, chopped
Salt and freshly ground black pepper

Steam the leek for 4–5 minutes or until tender, adding the courgette for the final 2 minutes. Set aside.

Using a small grinder, processor or pestle and mortar, make a paste with the ginger, chilli, garlic and lemon juice. Put the olive oil in a pan over a medium heat, tip in the paste and sauté for a couple of minutes.

Add the prawns and beans and sauté until the prawns are pink and cooked through, around 10 minutes. Add the leeks and courgette to the pan and toss together. Season with salt and pepper and then scatter over the chopped coriander before serving.

Trout on lime and coriander-crushed peas – 480 calories

Serves 2

Drizzle of olive oil
2 × 120g trout fillets
2 limes, 1 peeled and sliced and the other juiced
½ tsp ground cumin
200g frozen peas
1 tbsp Greek yoghurt
Large handful of coriander, finely chopped
Salt and freshly ground pepper

Preheat the oven to 180°C/gas mark 4. Lay the trout fillets in an ovenproof dish and drizzle with olive oil. Place the slices of lime on the fish, sprinkle with the cumin and season with salt and freshly ground black pepper. Roast the fish in the oven for 8 minutes or until cooked through.

Meanwhile, cook the peas in boiling water until tender. Drain, and place in a bowl, along with the yoghurt and lime juice. Use a potato masher to crush the peas into a coarse mash. Stir through most of the coriander and season with a pinch of salt and plenty of freshly ground black pepper.

Serve the trout on top of the mashed peas and sprinkle with the remaining coriander.

Lamb and pine nut meatballs with Moroccan salad – 480 calories
Serves 2

For the meatballs:
200g minced lamb
1 small onion, finely grated
2 garlic cloves, crushed to a paste
50g pine nuts, lightly toasted and roughly chopped
½ tsp paprika
¼ tsp ground allspice
½ tsp ground cumin
1 egg white, lightly whisked
Small bunch of fresh parsley, finely chopped
Small bunch of fresh mint, finely chopped
1 tbsp vegetable oil
Salt and freshly ground pepper

For the salad:
100g spinach leaves
1 tbsp sliced almonds
½ cucumber, peeled, seeded and cut into small chunks
2 tbsp chickpeas, drained and rinsed
2 spring onions, chopped
1 tsp olive oil
1 tbsp balsamic vinegar
Juice of half a lemon

In a large bowl, mix together the minced lamb, onion, garlic, pine nuts, paprika, allspice and cumin. Add the egg white and mix again. Stir in the chopped herbs and season to taste with salt and freshly ground black pepper. Shape the mixture into 6 evenly sized balls.

Heat the oil in a frying pan and fry the meatballs over a medium heat, turning occasionally, for 10 minutes, until golden brown on all sides and completely cooked through.

Place the spinach leaves in a bowl. Add all the other ingredients and toss together. Serve with the meatballs.

Pork with apples and shallots – 450 calories
Serves 8

1 boneless rolled pork leg joint (approx 3.5kg)
8 garlic cloves, crushed
1 bunch of fresh sage, finely chopped
5 tbsp olive oil
2 large leeks, diagonally sliced
16 shallots
6 small apples, cored and cut into quarters
1 tbsp butter
250ml cider

Preheat the oven to 240°C/gas mark 9. Unroll the pork and score the flesh with a sharp knife. Make a paste with the garlic, sage, a pinch of salt and pepper and 3 tbsp of the oil and then spread it over the meat. Roll the pork back up and tie it firmly.

Place the leeks in the bottom of a roasting dish, toss

with the remaining oil, then sit the pork on top and roast for about 25 minutes or until the skin has bubbled and crisped.

Meanwhile, in a frying pan, brown the shallots and apple wedges in the butter.

Turn the oven down to 180°C/gas mark 4. Place the shallots and apple wedges around the pork and roast for another 45 minutes to 1 hour, or until a meat thermometer reads 75–80°C.

Remove the pork, apples and shallots from the oven and keep warm. Strain the pan juices into a small saucepan, add the cider, bring to the boil and simmer until slightly thickened. Slice the pork and serve with the apples, shallots and gravy.

Spicy chicken and lentils – 470 calories
Serves 1

½ fennel bulb, thinly sliced
½ red onion, cut into thin wedges
1 garlic clove, crushed
Handful of fresh thyme
Drizzle of olive oil
Pinch of chilli flakes
1 skinless chicken breast
200ml vegetable stock
½ × 400g tin green lentils
50g mange tout

Preheat the oven to 200°C/gas mark 6. Place the fennel, onion wedges, garlic and thyme in a roasting tin, drizzle with a little olive oil and sprinkle on the chilli flakes. Place the chicken breast on top. Roast for 20 minutes, then remove from the oven and turn down the temperature to 150°C/gas mark 2.

Add the stock and lentils to the roasting tin and stir in around the chicken. Season well and then return the tin to the oven for another 20 minutes.

Meanwhile, steam or boil the mange tout for 3–4 minutes. Serve with the chicken and lentils.

Smoked mackerel and orange salad – 460 calories
Serves 2

200g small beetroots
2 tbsp red wine vinegar
Zest and juice of half an orange
1 tbsp olive oil
Pinch of salt and freshly ground black pepper
2 oranges
1 head of chicory
2 spring onions, sliced diagonally
2 small smoked mackerel fillets
20g walnut halves

Preheat the oven to 200°C/gas mark 6. Put the beetroot in a roasting tin with a couple of centimetres of water in the bottom. Cover with foil and roast in the oven for 30 minutes. Meanwhile put the oil, vinegar, orange juice and zest into a screw-top jar, season with salt and pepper and shake until well combined.

Remove the beetroots from the oven – they should be tender when pierced with a knife. When they are cool enough to handle, peel off the skins, top and tail them and then slice into rounds. Toss them in a little of the dressing.

Peel the oranges, following the contour of the fruit, then cut each one into thin slices. Trim the head of the chicory and separate the leaves, discarding the outer ones.

Arrange the leaves in a salad bowl and then add the sliced beetroot, orange rounds and spring onion. Flake the fish on top, add the walnuts and drizzle with the remaining dressing.

Griddled chicken on white bean mash – 440 calories
Serves 2

2 skinless chicken breasts
1 tbsp olive oil
Salt and black pepper
1 shallot, finely chopped
1–2 garlic cloves, chopped
1 × 400g tin cannellini beans, drained and rinsed
Large handful of flat-leaf parsley
Steamed green beans or broccoli to serve

Drizzle a little of the olive oil over the chicken breasts and season well with a pinch of salt and plenty of black pepper. Heat a griddle pan and cook the chicken breasts for 10 minutes, turning frequently.

Meanwhile, heat the remaining oil in a saucepan and add the shallots. Cook gently for 5 minutes, then add the garlic and cook for another 2 minutes until soft. Add the cannellini beans to the pan and mash roughly, adding a little stock or water to loosen. Stir in the parsley and season to taste.

Serve with the green veg.

Aubergine with lamb and pomegranate – 490 calories
Serves 2

2 aubergines, halved lengthways
1 tbsp olive oil
1 onion, finely chopped
½ tsp ground cumin
½ tsp paprika
½ tsp ground cinnamon
200g lean minced lamb
1 tbsp pine nuts
1 tbsp tomato purée
2 tbsp pomegranate seeds
Handful of flat-leaf parsley, chopped

Preheat oven to 220°C/gas mark 7. Place the aubergines in a roasting dish skin side down. Lightly smear with some of the olive oil, season with a pinch of salt and plenty of black pepper, and bake in the oven for 20 minutes.

Meanwhile, heat the remaining oil in a pan, add the onion and spices and cook over a medium heat for 8 minutes. Add the meat, pine-nuts and tomato purée and cook for a further 8 mins. Just before the end, stir in the pomegranate seeds.

Remove the aubergines from the oven and divide the lamb mixture evenly between each half. Return to the oven for a further 10 minutes. Serve topped with parsley leaves.

French fish stew – 390 calories
Serves 2

Drizzle of olive oil
1 shallot, finely chopped
1 fennel bulb, finely chopped
1 garlic clove, finely chopped
Splash of vermouth or dry white wine
300ml chicken stock
½ × 400g tin of chopped tomatoes
250g mixed fresh seafood (prawns, crab, white fish, crayfish, etc)
2–3 handfuls of spinach

Heat the oil in a large pan, add the shallot, fennel and garlic and cook for 5 minutes or until softened. Add the vermouth and let it bubble for a minute. Pour in the chicken stock and tomatoes and bring to the boil. Simmer for 15 minutes, then stir in the seafood and spinach and heat through. Season to taste.

Steak with crème fraîche and peppercorn sauce – 510 calories
Serves 2

200ml beef stock
100ml red wine
2 sirloin steaks (approx 225g each)
Pinch of steak seasoning/rub
1 tsp butter
1 tsp olive oil
2 tbsp crème fraîche
2 tsp mixed peppercorns, roughly crushed
2 large handfuls of mixed salad leaves

Pour the stock and wine into a small saucepan and boil rapidly for about 10 minutes to reduce it, then season with a pinch of salt.

Season the steaks with a pinch of steak seasoning or rub and allow to reach room temperature. Place the frying pan over a high heat and add the butter and oil. Keeping the heat high, fry the steaks for 3 minutes on one side for medium or 2 minutes for rare. Turn them over and give them another 2 minutes for medium or 1 minute for rare.

Pour in the reduced stock, crème fraîche and crushed

pepper. Stir well and cook for a further minute. Serve with a green salad.

Harissa chicken – 420 calories
Serves 2

2 skinless chicken breasts
4 tsp harissa paste
1 tbsp olive oil
1 tbsp pine nuts
4 large handfuls of baby spinach leaves
2 spring onions, chopped
¼ cucumber, chopped
2 tomatoes, chopped
200g haricot beans, drained and rinsed
1 tbsp raisins
Handful of flat-leaf parsley, chopped
Handful of mint, chopped

Preheat the oven to 180°C/gas mark 4. Smear each chicken breast with 2 tsp of the harissa paste and place in an ovenproof dish. Drizzle over the oil, season with salt and pepper and bake in the oven for 25 minutes or until cooked through. Remove from the oven, allow to cool slightly and then shred.

Put the pine nuts in a dry frying pan and place over a medium heat for a few minutes to toast – remove from the heat as soon as they turn golden as they can burn quickly.

Place the spinach leaves in a bowl and add the spring onions, cucumber, tomatoes, beans, raisins and herbs. Place the chicken on top and sprinkle with the pine nuts.

Crabcakes – 440 calories
Serves 1

100g crabmeat
1 tbsp tinned sweetcorn, drained and rinsed
Pinch of paprika
Splash of Worcestershire sauce
1 tsp mayonnaise
1 spring onion, chopped
Handful of parsley, chopped
Juice of half a lemon
Freshly ground black pepper
Flour for dusting
Drizzle of olive oil
A couple of broccoli florets

Mix together in a bowl the sweetcorn, crabmeat, paprika, Worcestershire sauce, spring onion, mayonnaise and parsley. Season and stir in the lemon juice. Place the bowl in the fridge for a few hours.

Sprinkle some flour, seasoned with black pepper, on a clean surface and on your hands and shape the mixture into 2 patties. Heat a little oil in a non-stick frying pan and when hot fry the crabcakes for 3 minutes on each side. Serve them with some steamed broccoli.

Foil-steamed fish – 370 calories
Serves 2

2 pieces skinless fish fillet (cod, haddock, etc), 120g each
2 tomatoes, chopped
4 spring onions, trimmed and cut on the diagonal
1 red chilli, deseeded and shredded
1 carrot, peeled and cut into julienne strips
Juice of 1 lime
1 tbsp soy sauce
Handful of fresh coriander, chopped
100g green beans

Preheat the oven to 220°C/gas mark 7. Place each fish fillet on a sheet of kitchen foil on a large baking tray. In a bowl, mix the tomatoes, spring onions, chilli and carrot, then pile half on top of each fish fillet. Drizzle the lime juice and soy sauce over them, and then wrap each fillet in the foil to make a parcel. Bake in the oven for 15 minutes.

Meanwhile, boil the green beans. Serve the fish with the beans, scattered with coriander.

Stir-fry 2 ways

Stir-fry chicken with lime and coconut milk – 340 calories
Serves 2

2 tsp rapeseed oil
2 skinless chicken pieces

1 green chilli, deseeded and finely chopped
150ml coconut milk
1 tbsp Thai fish sauce
Large handful of coriander, chopped
4 spring onions, chopped
Juice of 1 lime

Put the oil in a wok over a high heat, add the chicken pieces and stir-fry for 5 minutes, or until they're golden. Add the chilli, stir-fry for 1 minute, then add the coconut milk, fish sauce, coriander and spring onions. Cook for another 3 minutes, then serve, drizzled with the lime juice. You could serve with 2 tbsp cooked brown rice (adds 70 calories).

Gingered pork with stir-fried vegetables – 270 calories
Serves 2

1 tbsp soy sauce
2 tbsp red wine vinegar
2 garlic cloves, crushed
1 tbsp grated ginger
2 lean pork fillets (approx 125g each)
1 tsp rapeseed oil
1 medium onion, sliced
1 small carrot, finely sliced
1 courgette, sliced
2 tsp cornflour
150g mange tout, halved
100g bean sprouts

Combine the soy sauce, vinegar, garlic and ginger in a bowl, add the pork and mix well. Cover and refrigerate for several hours or overnight.

Preheat the oven to 180°C/Gas Mark 4. Drain the pork and reserve the marinade. Cook it in a non-stick pan until browned all over. Transfer to an ovenproof dish and bake in the oven for 30 minutes. Remove and slice diagonally.

Heat the oil in a wok, add the onion, carrot and courgette, and stir-fry over a high heat until tender. Blend the cornflour with the reserved marinade and a little water and add to the wok. Add the mange tout and bean sprouts, and stir until the sauce boils and thickens.

Serve with the pork and, if you want, 2 tbsp cooked brown rice (adds 70 cals).

Spicy turkey and apricot burgers with salad – 460 calories
Serves 2

For the burgers:
5 mushrooms
250g turkey mince
½ onion, finely chopped
6 dried apricots, finely chopped
1 tbsp flat-leaf parsley, finely chopped
1 tsp baharat spice mix
1 small egg, beaten

For the salad:
1 tbsp olive oil
3 spring onions, chopped
100g rocket leaves
50g blanched almonds
50g pomegranate seeds
100g cherry tomatoes, diced
Squeeze of lemon juice

Place the mushrooms in a food processer and blitz till they resemble breadcrumbs. Put all the rest of the ingredients for the burgers in a bowl, season with a pinch of salt and plenty of black pepper and mix together with your hands. Shape into evenly sized small balls.

Heat the oil in a frying pan and sear the burgers for 5 minutes or until browned all over, then turn down the heat and cook for another 10 minutes. Once cooked through, remove from the pan and keep warm. Using the same pan, fry the spring onions for 3 minutes.

Place the rocket in a bowl and toss with the cooked spring onions. Add the almonds, pomegranate and tomatoes and squeeze over some lemon juice and then serve with the burgers.

Braised cod with lettuce and peas – 440 calories
Serves 1

100g frozen peas

1 little gem lettuce, shredded
1 tbsp olive oil
140g boneless cod or white fish fillet
Salt and freshly ground black pepper
2 spring onions, thickly sliced
1 tbsp crème fraîche
Juice of half a lemon

Place the peas in a pan of boiling water and cook for 5 minutes. Add the lettuce and cook for a further 2 minutes. Drain well using a colander and then place the colander on top of the empty pan and put back on the heat for 1 minute; this allows the peas and lettuce to steam for a bit to remove any excess water.

Heat the olive oil in a large pan. Season the cod well and cook over a medium heat with the spring onions for 3–4 minutes each side.

Add the lettuce, peas, crème fraîche and lemon juice to the pan and gently heat through for a further 2 minutes.

Skinny chilli – 460 calories
Serves 8

500g mushrooms
2 tbsp rapeseed oil
500g beef mince
2 red onions, finely chopped
2 celery sticks, chopped
½–1 tbsp dried chilli flakes

½ tbsp ground cumin
½ tbsp dried oregano
2 × 400g tins chopped tomatoes
500ml beef or vegetable stock
1 x 400g tin kidney beans, drained and rinsed
1 x 400g tin black-eyed beans, drained and rinsed
1 cinnamon stick
Salt and freshly ground black pepper
75g plain chocolate, roughly chopped
Handful of fresh coriander, chopped
Greek yoghurt to serve

Preheat the oven to 150°C/gas mark 2. Place the mushrooms in a food processor and blitz till they resemble the
mince. Place half the oil in a large flameproof casserole
over a medium-high heat and add the beef mince. Fry
until browned all over then remove from the pan with a
slotted spoon and set aside. Add the remaining oil to the
pan and cook the onions and celery for 3–4 minutes. Stir
in the mushrooms, chilli flakes, cumin and oregano and
combine well. Cook for a further 3 minutes.

Return the mince to the pan, then stir in the tomatoes, stock, kidney beans and black-eyed beans. Snap the
cinnamon stick in half and add to the pan. Bring to the
boil, then reduce the heat and cover with a tight-fitting
lid. Place in the preheated oven and cook for 2–3 hours.

Remove from the oven and adjust the seasoning if
necessary. Add the chocolate pieces and stir until they
have just melted, then scatter over the chopped coriander.
Serve with the yoghurt.

QUICK AND EASY RECIPES

5-min breakfasts

Scrambled eggs 3 ways

Tomato and chive – 200 calories
Take 2 small eggs and whisk together in a bowl with a pinch of salt and plenty of black pepper. Heat a knob of butter in a pan and add the eggs. Use a spatula to push the eggs around the pan for 30 secs–1 min until cooked to your liking. Stir in a sprinkle of snipped chives and serve on a couple of thick slices cut from a beef tomato.

Creamy smoked salmon – 310 calories (brunch option)
Whisk a tbsp crème fraîche with 2 eggs, then pour into pan with 1 tsp of pre-melted butter. Add a sprinkle of chives and 50g of diced smoked salmon when the eggs are half-way done.

Chilli cheese – 230 calories
Scramble 2 eggs with ½ tsp finely chopped chilli. When the eggs are half-way done, add a handful of grated Parmesan cheese and continue cooking until done to your liking.

Cottage cheese 3 ways

Pear and walnuts – 210 calories
Spoon 100g cottage cheese into a bowl. Core and dice a small pear and stir into the cheese and scatter on a handful of chopped walnuts.

Middle Eastern – 90 calories
Spoon 100g cottage cheese into a bowl. Finely chop a tomato, a 5cm piece of cucumber and a handful of parsley. Stir into the cheese, add a squeeze of lemon juice and season with black pepper.

Raspberry and spinach – 140 calories
Spoon 100g cottage cheese into a bowl. Roughly chop a handful of baby spinach leaves and stir into the cheese. Add a handful of raspberries and gently crush into the cheese.

Avocado 3 ways

Poached egg –200 calories
Cut half an avocado into thick slices. Sprinkle with a pinch of paprika. Place a poached egg on top and season well.

Edam and pecans – 320 calories (brunch option)
Dice half an avocado. Place in a bowl and add a

matchbox-sized piece of Edam cheese, diced, and a handful of pecan nuts.

Tuna and spring onion – 200 calories
Put half an avocado in a bowl with a small tin of tuna, drained (the type in water, not oil), and a squeeze of lemon juice. Mash together and stir in a chopped spring onion. Serve on slices of beef tomato.

No-fuss lunches

Medi platter – 220 calories
Make up a platter with 2 tbsp any shop-bought hummus, a matchbox-sized piece of feta, a small handful of olives, 2–3 anchovies, a red pepper, a 7cm piece of cucumber cut into sticks, and a handful of halved cherry tomatoes.

Mexi platter – 350 calories
Make up a platter with 2 tbsp each of shop-bought guaca-mole, salsa and sour cream, 100g cooked chicken strips, and serve with a carrot and a celery stick cut into dipping sticks.

No-carb ploughman's – 290 calories

On a plate, place an apple, cored and cut into thick slices, with 2 sticks of celery, a matchbox-sized piece of Cheddar, 2 slices of ham, a handful of walnuts and a dollop of chutney (look for a low-sugar option rather than a sweet pickle).

Cheesy baked beans – 260 calories

Season 2 portobello mushrooms and place under the grill for 2 minutes. Heat half a tin of baked beans in a pan, add a splash of Worcestershire sauce and melt in a handful of grated mozzarella. Serve on the mushrooms.

Peanut butter dip – 230 calories

Mix 2 tbsp peanut butter with 1 tbsp soft cheese in a bowl. Cut a celery stick, a carrot, a 7cm piece of cucumber and a red pepper into sticks to dip.

Sardine dip – 320 calories

Mix 2 tbsp soft cheese with a small tin of drained sardines and a squeeze of lemon juice in a bowl. Season with plenty of black pepper and combine well. Cut a celery stick, a carrot, a 7cm piece of cucumber and a red pepper into sticks to dip.

Simple suppers

5 ways to jazz up a chicken breast

Lime and ginger – 130 calories:
Mix the juice from half a lime with ½ tsp 5-spice, a drizzle of olive oil, a splash of Thai fish sauce and 1 tsp ginger paste. Mix together and pour over the chicken. Pan-fry or bake in the oven.

Almond and basil –190 calories:
Finely chop a handful of basil leaves and place in a bowl with 1 tbsp each of ground almonds and grated Parmesan. Season and drizzle in a little olive oil. Mix together and spoon over the chicken and then bake in the oven.

Pepper and olive – 170 calories:
Finely chop 2 red peppers. Mix with a handful of finely chopped black olives and a pinch of chilli flakes. Spoon over the chicken with a drizzle of olive oil and bake in the oven.

Basil and pine nuts – 220 calories:
Place a handful of basil leaves in a food processor with 1 tbsp pine nuts, 1 tbsp grated Parmesan, salt and pepper and a drizzle of oil. Whizz together to make a pesto. Spoon over the chicken and bake in the oven.

Spinach and ricotta – 230 calories:
Place 2 tbsp ricotta in a bowl with a handful of finely chopped spinach leaves and 1 tbsp pine nuts. Make a slit lengthways along the chicken breast and spoon the mixture into the middle. Drizzle with oil and season and then bake in the oven.

3 ways to jazz up a salmon steak

Soy sauce and spring onion – 240 calories:
Mix the juice of a lemon with 1 tbsp each soy sauce and oyster sauce, 1 tsp grated ginger and a chopped spring onion.

Rub the mixture over a salmon steak and leave to marinate for an hour or so or overnight. When ready to cook, drain the fish and pan-fry, adding the remaining marinade for the last few minutes.

Lime and coriander – 200 calories:
Use a pestle and mortar to crush a handful of coriander leaves into the juice of a lime. Mix in ½ tsp ground cumin and a pinch of chilli flakes. Cover the salmon with the coriander mixture and pan-fry or bake in the oven.

Spicy sesame seed crust – 250 calories:
Mix 1 tbsp sesame seeds with a pinch of cayenne pepper and a squeeze of lemon juice. Place a salmon steak under

the grill and cook on one side. When ready to turn, spoon on the seed mixture and grill on the other side.

3 ways to jazz up a lamb chop

Mint – 170 calories:
Use a pestle and mortar to crush a handful of mint leaves into 1 tbsp each lemon juice and balsamic vinegar. Serve with a grilled lamb chop.

Mustard – 180 calories:
Crush a clove of garlic and mix with 2 tsp Dijon mustard and a handful of chopped rosemary leaves. Spread over a lamb chop before cooking.

Pecan crunch – 220 calories:
Gently crush together a handful of pecan nuts with 2 tsp lemongrass paste and a handful each of chopped thyme and parsley. Spread on the lamb before cooking.

3 ways with courgetti

Courgetti – 20 calories:
Allow 1 courgette per person. Use the large noodle attachment of a spiraliser to make the courgetti. Heat a drizzle of olive oil in a frying pan and cook the courgetti for

2–3 minutes or until softened and season with a pinch of salt and plenty of black pepper. Serve with any of the following:

Bolognaise – 260 calories:
(Makes 4 portions.) Heat a drizzle of olive oil in a large pan and add 1 tsp Italian herbs, a chopped red onion, a diced celery stick and a diced carrot. Gently sauté for 10 minutes. Add 400g lean beef mince and cook until evenly brown. Add a 400g tin of chopped tomatoes, 1 tbsp each tomato purée and Worcestershire sauce, and season well with a pinch of salt and plenty of black pepper. Bring to the boil, stir well and then cover and simmer for 1–1.5 hours.

Salmon and crème fraîche – 330 calories:
Mix 2–3 tbsp crème fraîche with 50g cooked flaked salmon and 2 tbsp cooked frozen peas and heat gently in a saucepan.

Arrabbiata – 150 calories:
(Makes 3 portions.) Heat a drizzle of olive oil in a pan, add 1 tsp each dried oregano and thyme, a chopped garlic clove, 1–2 crushed fresh chillies and the chopped stalks from a handful of basil leaves. Fry for a few minutes. Add a 400g tin of chopped tomatoes and 1 tbsp tomato purée. Simmer uncovered for about 8 minutes to let the excess water evaporate. Reduce the heat and cook for a few

more minutes, stirring occasionally. Add 1 tbsp balsamic vinegar, a pinch of salt and black pepper to taste and then stir in a handful of torn basil leaves.

3 ways with cauliflower "rice"

Cauliflower "rice" – 30 calories:
One cauliflower will serve 4. Cut the hard core and stalks from the cauliflower and pulse the rest in a food processor to make grains the size of rice. Then, either tip into a heat-proof bowl, cover with clingfilm, pierced in several places and microwave for 7 minutes on high – there is no need to add any water; or spread the cauliflower grains thinly on a baking tray and bake in a medium oven for 10–15 minutes. Stir in some chopped fresh coriander or toasted cumin seeds for flavour. Serve as:

Chicken and pea "pilaf" – 170 calories:
Heat a drizzle of oil in a pan and add 100g cooked chicken pieces and 2 tbsp cooked frozen peas. Cook until the peas have softened and then mix in the cauliflower rice.

Mushroom "risotto" – 210 calories:
Sauté 100g chopped mushrooms in a drizzle of olive oil and a tiny corner of butter. Add some chopped rosemary leaves and 30g diced goat's cheese and then mix in the cauliflower rice.

Veg curry – 270 calories:
(Makes 3 portions.) Heat a drizzle of oil in a large pan and add a chopped red onion and cook for 8 minutes or until softened. Add a diced courgette, a chopped red pepper, 100g chopped mushrooms and a small peeled and diced butternut squash. Mix in 2–3 tbsp curry paste of your choice and a 400g tin of chopped tomatoes. Bring to the boil, then simmer for 25–30 minutes, adding a splash of water if needed.

INSTANT SOUPS

Miso with baby veg – 70 calories:
Make up a miso soup from a sachet and add 2 handfuls of baby veg such as baby sweetcorn, sugar snap peas and mange tout.

Pho with cooked chicken and spinach – 130 calories:
Make up a pho base from a packet and add 100g cooked chicken and 2 large handfuls of spinach leaves.

Consommé with celeriac and spring onions – 40 calories:
Make up a consommé base and add 2 chopped spring onions and 80g grated celeriac.

GUILT-FREE BAKING

Courgette and pumpkin seed muffins – 170 calories each
Makes 12

3 tbsp butter
1 courgette
1 apple
Juice of 1 orange
4 large eggs
150g coconut flour
1 tsp baking powder
1 tsp mixed spice
50g pumpkin seeds

Preheat the oven to 220°C/gas mark 7. Line a muffin tray with muffin cases. Melt the butter in a small pan and set aside. Grate the courgette and apple into a bowl. Beat the egg and then stir into the grated courgette and apple. Add the orange juice and melted butter and mix well.

Sieve the flour and baking powder into a separate bowl, then gradually stir the wet mixture into the dry mixture until sticky and well combined. If the consistency still seems too dry and crumbly, add water, sparingly – a tbsp at a time – until it feels right. Stir in the pumpkin seeds.

Divide the mixture between the muffins cases. Bake in the oven for 12–15 minutes, or until a skewer inserted into the centre of the muffins comes out clean.

Cheesy scones – 180 calories each
Makes 12

175g coconut flour
6 tbsp butter
6 eggs
1 tsp baking soda
Pinch of salt
75g Cheddar, grated

Preheat oven to 200°C/gas mark 6 and line a baking tray with parchment paper. Tip all the ingredients into a food processor and pulse until blended. Allow the mixture to sit for 1–2 minutes so the dough expands. Shape into 12 evenly sized patties and press onto the baking tray. Bake for 15 minutes or until golden.

Guilt-free brownies – 120 calories each
Makes 16

4 tbsp coconut oil, melted
100g almond flour

Pinch of salt
½ tsp baking powder
100g cacao nibs
6 dates
3 large eggs

Preheat the oven to 180°C/gas mark 5 and, using a little of the coconut oil, grease a 20cm square baking tin. Mix all the ingredients together and transfer to the baking tin, smoothing over with a spatula. Bake for 20 minutes.

4-week menu plan

Things to note:

- Average daily intake – 800 calories (but remember, you do not have to adhere slavishly to the 800 mark: you are on this diet for a number of weeks, so the odd higher- or lower-cal day will quickly average out).

- Weekends are brunch, no lunch and a more substantial supper – but this is just a suggestion; you are welcome to treat them like normal weekdays.

- There is an option during the week to choose from the Quick and Easy section rather than the menu plan – just tot up the cal count yourself

Tip: try and have some sensible snacks handy – berries, almonds, hardboiled eggs, even a courgette and pumpkin seed muffin from the Guilt-free Baking list above – for those days when you are struggling. Much better one of these than that you reach for the biscuit tin!

Week 1

	Breakfast	Lunch	Dinner
Monday	Blueberry and green tea shake	Pepper with jewelled feta	Aubergine with lamb and pomegranate
Tuesday	Poached egg and avocado	No-carb ploughman's	Veg curry with cauli-flower rice
Wednesday	No-carb bircher	Beetroot falafels	Veg frittata
Thursday	Portobello 'toast' with goat's cheese and pine nuts	Sardine dip	Foil-steamed fish
Friday	Almond butter with apple and goji berries	Warm halloumi salad	Spicy chicken with lentils
Saturday	Cheesy baked beans		Steak with crème fraîche and peppercorn sauce
Sunday	Poached egg and salmon stack		Harissa chicken

Week 2

	Breakfast	Lunch	Dinner
Monday	Smoked salmon eggs	Hummus 3 ways	Chicken and Asparagus Salad
Tuesday	Yogurt with passion fruit and almonds	Beetroot, apple and cannellini bean soup	Luxury fish pie
Wednesday	Blueberry and green tea shake	Chicken and butter-bean salad	Crabcakes
Thursday	No-carb bircher	Lettuce cup	Griddled chicken on white bean mash
Friday	Portobello 'toast' with wilted spinach and chickpeas	Crayfish salad	Your choice from the "Quick and Easy" section
Saturday	Veg frittata		Skinny chilli
Sunday	No-carb waffles		Pork with apples and shallots

Week 3

	Breakfast	Lunch	Dinner
Monday	Avocado with tuna and spring onion	Chickpea and hazelnut salad	Courgetti prawns
Tuesday	Your choice from the "Quick and Easy"	Spanish chickpea and spinach soup	Stir-fry
Wednesday	Melon, spinach and blue-berry shake	Courgette and feta salad	French fish stew
Thursday	Your choice from the "Quick and Easy"	Lettuce cup	Harissa chicken
Friday	No-carb bircher	Grapefruit and Manchego salad	Braised cod with lettuce and peas
Saturday	Baked eggs with minted pea and feta salad		Lamb and pine nut meatballs with Moroccan salad
Sunday	Skinny kedgeree		Spicy turkey and apricot burgers

Week 4

	Breakfast	Lunch	Dinner
Monday	Yoghurt with rhubarb compote	Medi platter	Braised cod with lettuce and peas
Tuesday	Scrambled eggs with tomato and chive	Prawn pho	Smoked mackerel and orange salad
Wednesday	Yogurt with passionfruit and almonds	Chickpea and hazelnut salad	Courgetti prawns
Thursday	Your choice from "Quick and Easy"	Hummus 3 ways	Spicy chicken and lentils
Friday	Portobello 'toast' with goat's cheese and pine nuts	Chicken and asparagus salad	Your choice from "Quick and Easy"
Saturday	Mexican hash		Trout with coriander-crushed peas
Sunday	Poached egg and salmon stack		Aubergine with lamb and pomegranate

APPENDIX

The different types of diabetes

Type 1 diabetes is also known as "early onset" because it typically occurs in childhood, though it can occur later in life. For various reasons the body stops producing insulin, so type 1 diabetics have to get insulin by injections or via a pump. Although not closely linked to weight gain, keeping weight down and remaining active are still important

Type 2 diabetes is by far the most common form (90%) and used to occur mostly after the age of 40, though now it is starting to appear earlier and earlier. It happens when you become severely insulin-resistant or your pancreas stops producing enough insulin. There are many causes but high levels of fat in the liver and pancreas seem to be a major factor.

Gestational diabetes affects pregnant women. No one really knows why it happens but one theory is that hormones produced during pregnancy can block insulin receptors, making some women more insulin-resistant. It is important to test for the disease because it can affect the long-term health of mother and child. Babies who are exposed to high levels of glucose in the womb are more likely to become obese and develop diabetes later in life. In most women the insulin resistance goes soon after the child is born, but an Australian study found that 25% go on to develop diabetes within 15 years.[56]

Further blood measurements

HbA1c test

This is also known as the glycated haemoglobin or haemo-globin A1c test. Instead of measuring a single point in time (fasting glucose), this gives an estimate of your average blood sugar levels over the past few months.

Normal range:	Below 42mmol/mol (6.0%)
Prediabetes:	42 to 47mmol/mol (6.0–6.4%)
Diabetic:	Over 48mmol/mol (6.5%)

Why is HbA1c important? According to Diabetes UK, "People with diabetes who reduce their HbA1c by less than 1% can cut their risk of dying within five years by 50%."

The glucose tolerance test

This is a measure of how well your body is able to handle a big hit of sugar. After overnight fasting you have a blood test, are given a sugary drink, then have a series of blood tests over the next two hours. Initially your blood sugar will spike. At the end of two hours, however, it should have fallen back below 7.8mmol/l If not, you have problems.

Prediabetic: 7.9 to 11mmol/l
Diabetic: Over 11.0mmol/l

In pregnant women it is a concern if the two hour level is above 7.9mmol/l because of the increased risks for the baby.

NOTES

1. Prevalence of prediabetes in England from 2003 to 2011. A G Mainhous III et al, *British Medical Journal*, 2014. http://bmjopen.bmj.com/content/4/6/e005002.full
2. Prevalence and control of diabetes in Chinese adults. Xu Y et al. *Journal of the American Medical Association*, 2013. http://www.ncbi.nlm.nih.gov/pubmed/24002281
3. Increased consumption of refined carbohydrates and the epidemic of type 2 diabetes in the US. L Gross et al, *American Journal of Clinical Nutrition*, 2004. http://ajcn.nutrition.org/content/79/5/774.full
4. The Look Ahead Research Group, *New England Journal of Medecine*, 2013. http://www.nejm.org/doi/full/10.1056/NEJMoa1212914
5. Always hungry? Here's why. D Ludwig and M Friedman, *New York Times*, 2014. http://www.nytimes.com/2014/05/18/opinion/sunday/always-hungry-heres-why.html?_r=0
6. Effects of diet on metabolism in humans. D Ludwig, Harvard Medical School, 2012.
   High glycaemic foods, overeating, and obesity; D Ludwig et al. *Pediatrics*, 1999. 103:E26
7. Effects of diet on metabolism in humans. D Ludwig, Harvard Medical School, 2012.
8. Risk of cardiovascular and all-cause mortality in individuals with diabetes mellitus, impaired fasting glucose, and impaired glucose tolerance. E L Barr et al, Australian Diabetes, Obesity, and Lifestyle Study, 2007. http://www.ncbi.nlm.nih.gov/pubmed/17576864
9. Glucose tolerance status and risk of dementia in the community. T Ohara et al, *Neurology*, 2011, http://www.neurology.org/content/77/12/1126.abstract
10. Looking older: the effect of higher blood sugar levels. Leiden University Med Center, 2011. http://www.research.

leiden.edu/news/looking-older-blood-sugar-plays-a-role.
html

11. Who would have thought it? An operation proves to be the most effective therapy for adult-onset diabetes mellitus. W J Pories et al, *Annals of Surgery*, 1995. http://www.ncbi.nlm. nih.gov/pmc/articles/PMC1234815/

12. Type 2 diabetes: etiology and reversibility. R Taylor, *Diabetes Care*, 2013. http://care.diabetesjournals.org/ content/36/4/1047.short

13. Reappraisal of metformin efficacy in the treatment of type 2 diabetes: a meta-analysis of randomised controlled trials. R Boussageon et al, *Plos*, 2012. http://journals.plos.org/plos-medicine/article?id=10.1371/journal.pmed.1001204

14. Reversal of type 2 diabetes: normalisation of beta cell function in association with decreased pancreas and liver triacylglycerol. E L Lim, *Diabetologia*, 2011. http://www. ncbi.nlm.nih.gov/pubmed/21656330

15. Restoring normoglycaemia by use of a very low calorie diet in long- and short-duration type 2 diabetes. S Steven et al, *Diabet Med*, 2015. http://www.ncbi.nlm.nih.gov/ pubmed/25683066

16. *The Mind-Body Diabetes Revolution*, R Surwit, pub. Da Capo Press, 2005.

17. Ibid.

18. A single night of partial sleep deprivation induces insulin resistance in multiple metabolic pathways in healthy subjects. E Donga, et al, *Journal of Clinical Endocrinology & Metabolism*, 2010;95(6):2963-8. http://www.ncbi.nlm.nih. gov/pubmed/20371664

19. Systematic review and meta-analysis of different dietary approaches to the management of type 2 diabetes. O Ajala et al, *American Journal of Clinical Nutrition*, 2013. http:// www.ncbi.nlm.nih.gov/pubmed/23364002

20. Low carbohydrate diet to achieve weight loss and improve HbA1c in type 2 diabetes and prediabetes: experience from one general practice. D Unwin and J Unwin, *Practical Diabetes*, 2014. http://www.abc.net.au/catalyst/extras/

low%20carb/Low%20Carb%20Diet%20for%20Weight%20
Loss%20and%20Diabetes%20-%20Unwin%202014.pdf

21. Myths, presumptions, and facts about obesity. K Casazza
    et al, *New England Journal of Medecine*, 2013. http://www.
    nejm.org/doi/full/10.1056/NEJMsa1208051

22. The effect of rate of weight loss on long term weight
    management: a randomised controlled trial. K Purcell,
    University of Melbourne, *The Lancet/Diabetes &
    Endocrinology*, 2014. http://www.thelancet.com/journals/
    landia/article/PIIS2213-8587(14)70200-1/abstract

23. PREVention of diabetes through lifestyle Intervention and
    population studies in Europe and around the World. http//
    http://www.previewstudy.com/

24. The Minnesota starvation experiment. A Keys et al,
    University of Minnesota, 1944. http://www.apa.org/
    monitor/2013/10/hunger.aspx

25. Resting energy expenditure in short-term starvation is
    increased as a result of an increase in serum norepineph-
    rine. C Zauner et al, *American Journal of Clinical Nutrition*,
    2000. http://ajcn.nutrition.org/content/71/6/1511.full

26. Myths, presumptions, and facts about obesity. K Casazza
    et al, *New England Journal of Medecine*, 2013. http://www.
    nejm.org/doi/full/10.1056/NEJMsa1208051

27. Primary prevention of cardiovascular disease with a
    Mediterranean diet. R Estruch et al, *New England Journal
    of Medicine*, 2013. http://www.nejm.org/doi/full/10.1056/
    NEJMoa1200303#t=articleMethod

28. Standardised mindfulness-based interventions in health-
    care: an overview of systematic reviews and meta-analyses
    of RCTs. R A Gotink et al, *Plos*, 2015. http://journals.plos.
    org/plosone/article?id=10.1371/journal.pone.0124344

29. Primary prevention of cardiovascular disease with a
    Mediterranean diet. R Estruch et al, *New England Journal
    of Medicine*, 2013. http://www.nejm.org/doi/full/10.1056/
    NEJMoa1200303#t=articleMethod

30. The relationship between high-fat dairy consumption and
    obesity, cardiovascular, and metabolic disease. M Kratz et

al, *European Journal of Nutrition*, 2012. http://link.springer.com/article/10.1007%2Fs00394-012-0418-1

31. Effect of a high-fat Mediterranean diet on bodyweight. *The Lancet Diabetes & Endocrinology*, 2016; DOI: (10.1016/S2213-8587(16)30085-7)

32. Mediterranean diet may lower risk of diabetes. *American College of Cardiology*, 2014. http://www.sciencedaily.com/releases/2014/03/140327100806.htm

33. Mediterranean diet and invasive breast cancer risk among women at high cardiovascular risk in the PREDIMED trial. E Toledo et al, *JAMA*, 2015. http://archinte.jamanetwork.com/article.aspx?articleid=2434738&resultClick=

34. Adherence to a Mediterranean-Style Diet and Effects on Cognition. *Frontiers in Nutrition*, 2016. http://10.3389/fnut.2016.00022

35. Mediterranean diet improves cognition. E H Martinez-Lapiscina et al, *Journal of Neurology, Neurosurgery and Psychiatry*, 2013. http://jnnp.bmj.com/content/84/12/1318

36. Effects of initiating moderate alcohol intake on cardiometabolic risk in adults with type 2 diabetes. Y Gepner et al, *Annals of Internal Medicine*, 2015. http://annals.org/article.aspx?articleid=2456121

37. Diet and the prevention of cardiovascular disease: physicians' knowledge, attitudes, and practices. N Harkin et al, *Journal of the American College Cardiology*, 2015. http://content.onlinejacc.org/article.aspx?articleid=2198773

38. Low-fat diet not a cure-all. Harvard School of Public Health. http://www.hsph.harvard.edu/nutritionsource/low-fat/ Citing article: Low-fat dietary pattern and weight change over 7 years: the Women's Health Initiative Dietary Modification Trial. B V Howard et al, *Journal of the American Medical Association*, 2006.

39. Trends in mean waist circumference and abdominal obesity among US adults 1999-2012, E S Ford et al, *Journal of the American Medical Association*, 2014. http://jama.jamanetwork.com/article.aspx?articleid=1904816

40. Diabetes Prevention Program (DPP). http://www.niddk.nih.

gov/about-niddk/research-areas/diabetes/diabetes-preven-
tion-program-dpp/Pages/default.aspx

41. Reversal of type 2 diabetes: normalisation of beta cell
    function in association with decreased pancreas and liver
    triacylglycerol. E L Lim, *Diabetologia*, 2011. http://www.
    ncbi.nlm.nih.gov/pubmed/21656330

42. Restoring normoglycaemia by use of a very low calorie
    diet in long- and short-duration type 2 diabetes. S Steven
    et al, *Diabet Med*, 2015. http://www.ncbi.nlm.nih.gov/
    pubmed/25683066

43. The pull of the past: when do habits persist despite conflict
    with motives? D Neal et al, USC, *Personality and Social
    Psychology Bulletin*, 2011. http://www.feinberg.north-
    western.edu/sites/ipham/docs/WW_WIP20130122_Habits.
    pdf

44. Slim by design: kitchen counter correlates of obesity. B
    Wansink et al, Cornell Univ, *SSRN*, 2015.

45. Are breaks in self-weighing associated with weight gain?
    E E Helander et al, *Plos*, 2014. http://journals.plos.org/
    plosone/article?id=10.1371/journal.pone.0113164

46. The effect of intermittent energy and carbohydrate restric-
    tion v. daily energy restriction on weight loss and metabolic
    disease risk markers in overweight women. M Harvie et al,
    British Journal of Nutrition, 2013. http://www.ncbi.nlm.nih.
    gov/pubmed/23591120

47. Does exercise without weight loss improve insulin sensi-
    tivity? R Ross, *Diabetes Care*, 2003

48. Coronary heart disease and physical activity of work. J N
    Morris, *Lancet* 265, 1053-1057, 1953.

49. Sedentary time in adults and the association with diabetes,
    cardiovascular disease and death: systematic review and
    meta-analysis. EG Wilmot et al, *Diabetologia*, 2012

50. Television viewing time and reduced life expectancy: a
    life table analysis. J L Veerman et al, *British Journal of
    Sports Medicine*, 2012. http://www.ncbi.nlm.nih.gov/
    pubmed/23007179

51. Interrupting prolonged sitting impacts blood sugar

metabolism. M C Peddie et al, *American Journal of Clinical Nutrition*, 2013.

52. Standing-based office work shows encouraging signs of attenuating post-prandial glycaemic excursion. J P Buckley et al. University of Chester, 2013. http://oem.bmj.com/content/early/2013/12/02/oemed-2013-101823.full.pdf?keytype=ref&ijkey=fvcEm117fzTcT51

53. The effects of free-living interval-walking training on glycemic control, body composition, and physical fitness in type 2 diabetic patients: a randomized, controlled trial. K Karstoft et al, *Diabetes Care*, 2013. http://www.ncbi.nlm.nih.gov/pubmed/23002086

54. High-intensity circuit training using bodyweight: Maximum Results With Minimal Investment. B Klika et al. *ACSM'S Health & Fitness Journal*, 2013. http://journals.lww.com/acsm-healthfitness/fulltext/2013/05000/high_intensity_circuit_training_using_body_weight_.5.aspx

55. Neural correlates of mindfulness meditation-related anxiety relief. F Zeidan et al, *Social Cognitive and Affective Neuroscience*, 2013. http://scan.oxfordjournals.org/content/early/2013/06/03/scan.nst041.full.pdf

56. Gestational diabetes mellitus: clinical predictors and long-term risk of developing type 2 diabetes: a retrospective cohort study using survival analysis, A J Lee et al, *Diabetes Care*, 2007. http://www.ncbi.nlm.nih.gov/pubmed/17392549

INDEX

kidney beans
  blood sugar diet 121
  skinny chilli 239–40
  skinny spicy bean burgers 217–18
kidney disease 47
Kratz, Dr Mario 116

LaBelle, Patti 21
lamb
  3 ways to jazz up a chop 247
  aubergines with lamb and pomegranate
    230–1
  lamb and pine nut meatballs with
    Moroccan salad 225–6
Last Chance Diet 98–100
Lean, Prof Mike 68, 102–3
leeks, pork with apple and shallots 226–7
legumes 85, 116, 118, 121
lentils
  blood sugar diet 121
  Glycaemic Load (GL) 94
  Mediterranean diet 85
  spicy chicken and lentils 227–8
lettuce
  braised cod with lettuce and peas
    238–9
  lettuce cups 3 ways 206
life expectancy 47, 58, 74
lifestyle changes 155–62, 168–73
lime and ginger chicken 245
Linn, Robert 98–9
lipid profile 130
lipoprotein lipase (LPL) 51–2
liquid diets 98–100
liver
  alcohol intake 142
  fat loss 110
  fat storage 9, 10, 54–5, 95, 142
  fructose 95
  MRI scans 65–6
  stress 181
  tests 130, 131
Look Ahead trial 34
Lorna (case study) *see* Norman, Lorna
low-fat diets 20, 33–4, 38, 84, 115, 123
Ludwig, Dr David 37–8
lunch platters 243–4
Lustig, Dr Robert 36–7

M Plan 111–12, 115–23 *see also*
  Mediterranean diet
M score 117–18
mackerel
  skinny kedgeree 204–5
  smoked mackerel and orange salad
    228–9
maintenance programmes 102–3, 153,
  155–65
mango 122
  breakfast yoghurt 193
margarine 122
Marshall, Dr Barry 59–61
Martin, Dr Corby 101–2
Maudsley, Henry 79
Mayer, Jean 35
meal plans 138
meal-replacement foods 63, 136–7
meals
  restaurants 159–60
  sitting down 156
meat, processed 116, 118, 122
meatballs, lamb and pine nut meatballs
  with Moroccan salad 225–6
Medi platter 243
medication
  diabetes 22, 58–9, 61, 70
  doctor's advice before starting diet
    67–8, 77, 124–5
meditation 114 *see also* mindfulness
Mediterranean diet 85, 111–12, 115–23,
  138
melon 118, 122
  melon, spinach and blueberry shake
    198
menu plans 256–9
metabolic rates 104–5
metabolic syndrome 21, 91
metformin 58–9, 61, 70, 124
Mexi platter 243
Mexican hash 203
Middle Eastern cottage cheese 242
mindfulness 114, 156, 183–7
mindset 182–3
miso soup with baby veg 250
monitoring progress 126–7, 129, 153,
  155, 164
Monroe, Marilyn 129
mood changes 39–40, 78–9, 81, 82–3, 149

ABOUT THE AUTHOR

Michael Mosley trained to be a doctor at the Royal Free Hospital in London. After qualifying he joined the BBC, where he has been a science journalist, executive producer and, more recently, a well-known television presenter. He has won numerous television awards, including an RTS, and was named Medical Journalist of the Year by the British Medical Association. He is the author of two books, *The Fast Diet*, co-written with Mimi Spencer (Short Books, 2012), and *Fast Exercise* (Short Books, 2013). He is married to a doctor and has four children, amongst them a son who is at medical school.

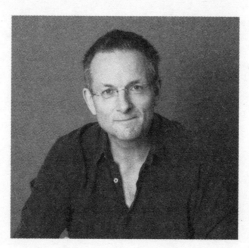